Springer Series on
Behavior Therapy and Behavioral Medicine

Series Editors: Cyril M. Franks, Ph.D., and Frederick J. Evans, Ph.D.

Advisory Board: John Paul Brady, M.D., Robert P. Liberman, M.D., Neal E. Miller, Ph.D., and Stanley Rachman, Ph.D.

Patrick J. McGrath, Ph.D. is senior psychologist in the behavioral program in the psychology department at the Children's Hospital of Eastern Ontario. He is principal investigator on research projects studying childhood migraine, recurrent abdominal pain, and compliance to hearing aid use. Other research interests include hyperactivity, pediatric compliance, and chronic pain in children.

Dr. McGrath completed his Ph.D. at Queen's University, Kingston, Ontario in 1979. He taught at the University of Regina, Saskatchewan, before assuming his present position in 1980. Dr. McGrath's extensive clinical practice is in behavioral medicine and behavior therapy with families. He is active in teaching special education teachers, psychology graduate students, medical residents, and day care workers.

Recently, in order to encourage his research in behavioral medicine, a Career Scientist Award was presented by the Ontario Ministry of Health to Dr. McGrath.

Philip Firestone, Ph.D. received his doctorate in clinical psychology from McGill University, Canada, in 1974. From that time until 1979 he was in the department of psychology at the Children's Hospital of Eastern Ontario. His primary interests are in the behavioral approach to the treatment of childhood psychopathology and family discord, and in behavioral medicine.

Dr. Firestone is presently an associate professor in the School of Psychology and Director of the Child Study Centre. In addition, he is a consultant to the department of psychology at the Children's Hospital of Eastern Ontario.

Pediatric and Adolescent Behavioral Medicine
Issues in Treatment

Patrick J. McGrath, Ph.D.
Philip Firestone, Ph.D.
Editors

Foreword by Frederick J. Evans, Ph.D.

Springer Publishing Company
New York

Springer Publishing Company, Inc.
200 Park Avenue South
New York, New York 10003

83 84 85 86 87 / 10 9 8 7 6 5 4 3 2 1

Library of Congress Cataloging in Publication Data

Main entry under title:

Pediatric and adolescent behavioral medicine.

(Springer series on behavior therapy and behavioral
medicine; 10)
  Includes bibliographies and index.
  1. Pediatrics—Psychological aspects—Congresses.
2. Youth—Diseases—Psychological aspects—Congresses.
3. Sick children—Psychology—Congresses.   4. Behavior
therapy—Congresses.   I. McGrath, Patrick J.   II. Firestone, Philip.   III. Series   [DNLM: 1. Behavior therapy
—In infancy and childood.   2. Behavior therapy—In
adolescence.   W1 SP685NB   v.10 / WS 350.6 P3702]
RJ47.5.P3   1982   618.92'0001'9   82-16734
ISBN 0-8261-4010-6
ISSN 0278-6729

Printed in the United States of America

To Chuck, a dear friend and teacher

—PM

To Suzie

—PF

Contents

Foreword

This outstanding collection is concerned with the interface of behavioral medicine and traditional primary care pediatrics. The burgeoning new field of behavioral medicine has already had an important impact on adult health care. This book will help lead to a clear recognition that the principles of behavioral medicine are as readily applicable to children and adolescents as they are to adults. As in adult medicine, specialization in pediatrics often leads to superior clinical care of specific diseases, syndromes, and symptoms, but the demands of specialization place undue burdens on the specialized practitioner and the primary care physician. Pediatricians and researchers interested in children's health need to recognize the interdisciplinary nature of all illness, and the significance of the context in which sick people, adult and child alike, must interact. Especially in pediatrics, behavioral issues are often central as the suffering child interacts with the family and the health care system. The practicing pediatrician spends a considerable amount of time and energy on the behavioral, social, and psychological impact of illness on the child and family, but unfortunately he/she is not always well equipped to deal with these special complex problems.

Parents bring children to pediatricians for relatively clear-cut reasons: Apart from preventive medicine, these presenting "symptoms" almost always include combinations of fever, specific medical symptoms, fear and anxiety (parent and/or child), pain and suffering, and behavioral problems. Add the iatrogenic effects of the treatment process itself and it seems evident that the increasing specialization that leads to superior treatment of specific symptoms must necessarily be accompanied by decreased ability, because of time and training, to adequately manage the nonspecific problems. Not surprisingly, bedside manner is being replaced by behaviorism at the bedside. This process itself has been painful and anxiety provoking, as evidenced by a variety of subspecialties in pediatrics that are outgrowths of early attempts to grapple with this void in clinical knowledge. The present contributions to pediatric behavioral medicine suggest that the field is developmentally approaching its adolescence.

The editors have clarified for us subtle distinctions between medical psychology, pediatric psychology, behavioral pediatrics, and pediatric behavioral medicine. With skill they have selected contributors who focus clearly on the new field by virtue of their clinical sensitivity and research experience. The body of knowledge providing the foundation for a developing field is necessarily sparse, and recent findings often have not been replicated and applied to clinical practice. For this reason, the topics selected for review are mere samples of the potential domain of pediatric behavioral medicine. Were I to edit such a volume I also would have sought, for example, material on children with cancer, childhood sleep disorders, drug and alcohol addiction, hyperactivity and so on; such topics must wait. This merely attests to the breadth of this new field and does not detract from the in-depth coverage of the eight areas that are represented in this book. Certainly the clinician will have some of his cherished assumptions challenged in the chapters on abdominal pain and asthma. He will be surprised at the extent of our knowledge about blood pressure elevation and reactivity in children. Exciting new clinical techniques that can be adapted to office practice will be learned concerning childhood obesity and adolescent cigarette smoking. Hospitalization and patient compliance are major issues in pediatrics, and the clinician will find the contributions in these areas to be especially rewarding and comprehensive.

The editors of this book have provided a major service for those who treat children and adolescents by placing difficult medical problems in their full behavioral and medical frameworks. In doing so, a number of conventional wisdoms have been challenged in a way that will provide vastly improved health care delivery for those practitioners who take the time to study the book. More important, by helping to delineate a new field of study, the clinical researcher in these fields will have a new baseline against which existing current knowledge can be properly evaluated, and will quickly become aware of those important areas that require additional empirical work.

Frederick J. Evans, Ph.D.
Carrier Foundation
UMDNJ—Rutgers Medical School
Belle Mead, N.J.

Preface

Although numerous health disciplines have been related historically to medicine, a pronounced increase in the contribution of nonmedical sciences to improved health care has been seen in recent years. In the behavioral sciences, the appearance of new journals (*Biofeedback and Self Regulation, Journal of Behavioral Medicine, Pediatric Psychology*) and professional societies (Society of Behavioral Medicine, Society of Pediatric Psychology) is evidence of this trend. Family physicians and pediatricians have long recognized that the problems of many of the children and adolescents whom they treat have a considerable behavioral component. As well, the increased collaboration of behavioral and medical scientists in health care and research is due to the recognition of the need to treat the whole child in context and not simply isolated aspects of the child. Finally, it has become evident that the delivery of medical services may be more effective and efficient and the iatrogenic aspects of medical care may be reduced with behavioral science input.

This book is concerned with the interface between behavioral science and traditional medical care for children and adolescents. Nevertheless, the title, *Pediatric and Adolescent Behavioral Medicine*, requires some explanation. We believe that it is important to describe and delineate the relationships among behavioral medicine, medical psychology, pediatric and adolescent psychology, behavioral pediatrics, and pediatric and adolescent behavioral medicine.

Schwartz & Weiss (1978), at the Yale Conference on Behavioral Medicine in 1977, produced a generally accepted definition of the term "behavioral medicine." It is

> [t]he interdisciplinary field concerned with the development and integration of behavioral and biomedical science knowledge and techniques relevant to health and illness and the application of this knowledge and these techniques to prevention, diagnosis, treatment and rehabilitation. [p. 250]

Behavioral medicine is interdisciplinary, by definition, and not a subspeciality of any one profession. Pediatric and adolescent behavioral medicine is that part of behavioral medicine focusing on children, adolescents, and their families.

Bradley & Prokop (1981) suggest that medical psychology, on the other hand, may focus on the same areas as other medical specialities; however, it is unique in its "assessment approach and its capability to provide empirical evaluation of diagnostic, preventative and treatment methods" (p. 4). In particular they describe medical psychologists as specialists trained in "(1) the assessment of brain–behavior relationships, (2) the construction of psychometric instruments and interpretation of patients' responses to these instruments; and (3) the functional analysis of behavior that encompasses measurement of overt and covert controlling stimuli. . . ." (p. 3).

Pediatric psychology may be seen as the specialty of medical psychology for children. The unique characteristics of pediatric psychology include (1) its emphasis on developmental evaluation, (2) its consultation in child rearing, (3) its short-term treatment, and (4) the study of normal personality or positive mental health (Tuma, 1980). Behavioral pediatrics, on the other hand, can be seen as part of the medical specialty of pediatrics that stresses the "bio-social, psychologic and developmental aspects" of children (Green, 1980–81). Behavioral pediatrics is an area of research and care for pediatricians and other physicians who are primary-care providers. Adolescent medicine is the medical specialty that deals with the medical and psychosocial problems of adolescents. All of pediatric psychology and behavioral pediatrics and those areas of medical psychology that deal with children and their families can be subsumed under the more general interdisciplinary classification of pediatric and adolescent behavioral medicine.

This volume came about as the result of a conference held in Ottawa, Canada in May 1981, designed for practitioners and researchers who work with children and their families. The contributors to this book presented their papers at that conference. In Chapter 1, Edward Christophersen focuses on the office practice of pediatricians and details how behavioral medicine approaches can help make the daily office routine more effective without sacrificing efficiency. Chapter 2 addresses the perplexing problem, in children, of recurrent abdominal pain of no known organic origin and presents evidence that the predominant psychogenic view may well be in error. The authors, Ronald Barr and Michael Feuerstein, point out that this psychogenic view may be a gross disservice to our patients and their families and contribute to the problems these children have. Similarly, in Chapter 3, Barney Alexander carefully reviews the literature on asthma to provide a most convincing argument that psychogenic factors have a very limited role in our understanding of asthma.

Thomas Coates' chapter on elevated blood pressure in adolescents (Chapter 4) is a challenge for all who have not considered the implications of early detection and treatment of one of our most serious health problems, high blood pressure. In Chapter 5, Belinda Traughber and Michael Cataldo have taken a unique approach to the issue of the hospitalization of children. They have grounded their intervention approach firmly in the experimental animal literature and as a result have provided new insights. Chapter 6, by Brian Flay and his associates, includes both a comprehensive review of the reasons why children smoke and an outline of an exciting and effective program that describes how to prevent smoking in adolescents.

Kelly Brownell and Albert Stunkard are names that we normally associate with careful research on adult obesity. In Chapter 7 they outline very promising work that has been done on childhood obesity. The last chapter, by Jacqueline Dunbar, is, most appropriately, on compliance, a problem that plagues all practitioners and challenges the researcher.

We wish to thank the Children's Hospital of Eastern Ontario and the University of Ottawa for financial and moral support. In particular, we appreciated the support and encouragement of Dr. J. Goodman, Director of the Department of Psychology at the Children's Hospital. Madeleine Gosselin carried the greatest burden, most cheerfully and efficiently, in organizing the conference and preparing the manuscript for publication.

Numerous others assisted in many different aspects of the conference and this volume. These include Clare Ball, Elisabeth Bartoli, Carol Bentivoglio, Anne Caron, June Cunningham, Anne Johnson, Francine Lafrance, Kevin McGrath, Mary-Jean McGrath, Sue Nigra, Joan Oliver, Sue Peters, Claire Thivièrge, Conny Withers, Jody Witt, Media Services, and Margaret Taylor and the library staff of the Children's Hospital of Eastern Ontario.

Patrick J. McGrath
Philip Firestone
Ottawa

References

Bradley, L. A., & Prokop, C. K. The relationship between medical psychology and behavioral medicine. In L. A. Prokop & C. K. Bradley (eds.), *Medical psychology: Contributions to behavioral medicine*. New York: Academic Press, 1981.

Green, M. The Pediatric model of health care. *Behavioral Medicine Update,*
  1980–81, 2:4, 11–15.
Schwartz, G. E., & Weiss, S. M. Behavioral medicine revisited: An Amended
  definition. *Journal of Behavioral Medicine,* 1978, 1:3, 249–251.
Tuma, J. M. Training in pediatric psychology: A concern of the 1980's. *Journal of
  Pediatric Psychology,* 1980, 5:3, 229–243.

Contributors

A. Barney Alexander, Ph.D., 8790 West Colfax Avenue, Suite 105, Denver, Colorado 80215

Ronald G. Barr, MDCM, FRCP(C), The Montreal Children's Hospital and McGill University, 2300 Tupper Street, Montreal, Quebec H3H 1P3

J. Allan Best, Ph.D., Department of Health Studies, University of Waterloo, Waterloo, Ontario N2L 3G1

Kelly D. Brownell, Ph.D., Department of Psychiatry, University of Pennsylvania, 205 Piersol Building, Philadelphia, Pennsylvania 19104

Michael F. Cataldo, Ph.D., John F. Kennedy Institute and Johns Hopkins University School of Medicine, 707 North Broadway, Baltimore, Maryland 21205

Edward R. Christophersen, Ph.D., University of Kansas Medical Center, 39th Street at Rainbow Boulevard, Kansas City, Kansas 66103

Thomas J. Coates, Ph.D., The Johns Hopkins Medical Hospital, 600 North Wolfe Street, Baltimore, Maryland 21205

Josie R. d'Avernas, M.Sc., Department of Health Studies, University of Waterloo, Waterloo, Ontario N2L 3G1

Jacqueline Dunbar, Ph.D., Psychiatric and Behavioral Sciences, Stanford University, Stanford, California 94305

Michael Feuerstein, Ph.D., Department of Psychology, McGill University, 2300 Tupper Street, Montreal, Quebec H3H 1P3

Brian R. Flay, D. Phil., Health Behavior Research Institute, University of Southern California, 1985 Zonal Avenue, Los Angeles, California 90033

Mary W. Kersell, M.Sc., Department of Health Studies, University of Waterloo, Waterloo, Ontario N2L 3G1

Katherine B. Ryan, B.A., Department of Health Studies, University of Waterloo, Waterloo, Ontario N2L 3G1

Albert J. Stunkard, M.D., University of Pennsylvania School of Medicine, 205 Piersol Building, Philadelphia, Pennsylvania 19104

Belinda Traughber, Ph.D., Rutherford County Guidance Centre, P.O. Box 1559, Murfreesboro, Tennessee 37130

CHAPTER 1

Behavioral Pediatrics: An Overview

Edward R. Christophersen, Ph.D.

Virtually all persons working with children, regardless of their research or clinical focus, have been able to refer to their work as behavioral pediatrics. There is no subspecialty area in pediatrics that is called *behavioral pediatrics;* the actual definition of the area undoubtedly will evolve over a period of time. The professions of child psychiatry and clinical child psychology exist, among other reasons, to deal in depth with children who present with significant psychopathology. Whether inpatient or outpatient, both psychiatry and psychology have developed procedures for the treatment of disturbed and seriously disturbed children. Whether the presenting problems are purely behavioral or are medical/behavioral, calling upon a psychiatrist or psychologist for assistance in assessment, evaluation, and development of a treatment plan is well precedented.

What, then, is the province of behavioral pediatrics? Is this a duplication of the efforts already put forth by professionals outside of pediatrics, or is this—in fact as well as in practice—a new area within the domain of pediatrics? What follows is a discussion of several different ways of approaching the actual practice of behavioral pediatrics from the perspective of the full-time primary-health-care provider. Obviously, with the pediatrician[1] maintaining responsibility for each child's primary care, an analysis of how pediatricians typically spend their time and of the types of problems seen will affect their ability to incorporate behavioral pediatrics into an already busy schedule.

Preparation of this manuscript was supported in part by a grant from NICHD (HD 03144) to the Bureau of Child Research, University of Kansas. The editorial assistance of Barbara Cochrane is gratefully acknowledged.

[1]Throughout this chapter, the generic term *pediatrician* will be used to refer to pediatricians, child health associates, nurse clinicians, or family practitioners who deliver primary care to pediatric-age patients.

1

Pediatric Practice

The Task Force on Pediatric Education (1978) estimated that there are currently approximately 22,000 full-time equivalent pediatricians in general pediatric practice in the United States. These pediatricians work, on the average, 240 days per year, seeing an average of 27 patients per day in order to meet the current demands for pediatric care. According to Bergman, Dassel, & Wedgwood (1966), the general pediatrician's day is broken down as follows:

Percentage of Day

With Patients	Telephone	Consulting	Paper Work	Auto Travel	Foot Travel	Other
48%	12.5%	8%	8%	4%	2%	7%

In this same paper, Bergman et al. calculated that the average pediatric office visit lasted a total of 11 minutes across all categories of care, with slightly more (13 minutes) devoted to well-child care. The authors stated that approximately 50 percent of the pediatrician's time and 46 percent of the patient load was spent in well-child care; another 22 percent of the time (or 27 percent of the patient load) was devoted to the diagnosis and management of respiratory infections. These figures are essentially the same as those quoted by Starfield (1980), which were taken from the National Center for Health Statistics' 1975 report, "Office Visits to the Pediatrician." According to Reisinger & Bires (1980), these figures for the average time devoted to well-child visits do not vary appreciably when consideration is given either to the type of practice (group, partnership, or solo) or to the number of years the individual pediatrician has been in practice (4–13, 14–23, or 24–27 years).

From the perspective of the full-time general pediatrician, one might argue that the first priority of behavioral pediatrics should be to address such issues as how to provide comprehensive as well as cost- and time-effective well-child care. Since the average pediatrician spends only 10 to 15 minutes with each patient/parent, this time must be highly structured in order to be productive. Behavioral pediatrics can make a substantial contribution by developing a variety of organizational protocols or packages to aid pediatricians in their delivery of well-child care. Christophersen & Rapoff (1979) rely heavily on the use of a flowchart that is designed to be affixed permanently to each child's medical chart. As items of well-child care are completed, they are checked off or dated, thereby replacing much of the need to refer to previous narrative charting for each office visit.

Anyone in the physician's office can glance at the flowchart and ascertain exactly how up-to-date the child's well-child care is. A similar system has been described by McConnochie (1980).

A related issue concerns the amount of time that the pediatrician devotes to the well-child physical examination, which was mentioned by Starfield (1980) as constituting almost 30 percent of the office visits. Leake, Barnard, & Christophersen (1978) examined the completeness of the well-child physical examinations as performed by first-year pediatric residents. During a baseline (or pre-education) phase, these residents were completing only 52 percent of what they consensually agreed was the minimum well-child physical. With the introduction of an education feedback package, the residents' completeness score was increased to an average of 85 percent.

One component of this educational feedback package was a single-page summary of all the maneuvers that constitute an acceptable well-child physical examination. This one-page summary, presented in Figure 1.1, now is used in the pediatric clerkship (for medical students) to assist medical students in their attempts to learn how to conduct a thorough well-child physical efficiently. The performance of such a physical can be conceptualized as *response chaining;* that is, each physical that the physician performs should have the maneuvers done in exactly the same sequence in order to lessen the probability that any of the maneuvers will be omitted inadvertently. The medical student can be instructed to begin a physical examination with the maneuver on the top left, proceeding down each column, and across each row, checking off each maneuver as it is completed. Initially, most students probably will need to refer to the chart after each maneuver. Later, as their proficiency improves, they need only check off each category (for example, "cardiovascular") as the requisite maneuvers are completed. Later still, each column can be checked off when all of the maneuvers contained therein are completed. Ultimately, the student will need the chart only at the end of an examination, as a final check to make sure that no maneuver was omitted.

Morbidity and Mortality

A second method for prioritizing pediatric care is to concentrate on health education efforts to reduce morbidity and/or mortality of young children. According to Starfield (1980), after the newborn period the greatest threat to life and limb is presented by accidents, which accounted for over 35,000 deaths in the United States in 1975, with vehicular accidents rating number one and burns as number two.

Figure 1.1   Physical Exam Check Sheet

Physician _____   Patient _____

Cardiovascular
Inspection
  Undressed ____
  Stethoscope Warmed ____
Pulses   L   R
  Femoral   ___ ___
Auscultation
  Mitral ____
  Tricuspid ____
  Pulmonary ____
  Aortic ____

Pulmonary
Inspection
  Undressed ____
Auscultation   L   R
  Ant Thorax   ___ ___
  Post Thorax   ___ ___

Abdomen
Inspection
  Undressed ____
Palpation
                        L   Mid   R
Inf   ___   ___ ___
Mid   ___   ___ ___
Sup   ___   ___ ___

Genitalia
Inspection
  Undressed ____
Palpation
  Male
    Elevates shaft of penis ____
                               L   R
    Palpates scrotum   ___ ___
    Spreads buttocks to
      observe anus ____
  Female
    Spreads labia ____
    Spreads buttocks to observe anus ____

Hips
Check for dislocation ____

Spine
Manually palpated sacral area ____

Head
Check fontanel ____
Measure H.C. ____
Manually inspect scalp ____

Eyes
                                      L   R
Red reflex   ___ ___
Pupillary reflex   ___ ___
Scanning ____

Ears
Otoscope held properly ____
                                      L   R
Grasp pinna and insert speculum ___ ___
Manually inspect pinna   ___ ___

Mouth
                                      L   R
Insert tongue blade   ___ ___
Check buccal mucosa   ___ ___

Neck
Supple ____
Nodes   L   R
  Post   ___ ___
  Ant   ___ ___
  Pre-auricular area   ___ ___
  Post-auricular area   ___ ___

Neuro-Growth and Development
Birth–1 mo.
  Pull to sit ____
  Ventral suspension ____
  Moro ____
  Suck ____
  Palmar grasp ____
  Smiles ____
  Follows to midline ____
1 mo.–5 mos.
  Lift head ____
  Smiling ____
  Rolls over ____
  Reaches ____
  Babbles ____
6 mos.–1 yr.
  Sits alone ____
  Crawls ____
  Stands ____
  Cruises ____
  Walks ____
  Speech ____
  DTR ____

Legend
____ = Couldn't observe
____ = Performed
____ = Not performed

Automobile Accidents

Numerous articles over the past decade have detailed efforts by pediatricians to reduce the risk of automobile accidents by encouraging parents or guardians to purchase and use child-restraint seats correctly. Although initial attempts were not very successful (e.g., Pless, 1978), several more recent articles have presented data describing compliance rates that exceed 50 percent. Reisinger, Williams, Wells, John, Roberts, & Podgainy (1981) obtained some of the highest correct car-seat usage rates by combining several components: (1) discussion during obstetrics hospitalization between the new mother and her pediatrician regarding the hazards of automobile travel; (2) pamphlets given to parents detailing the hazards of automobile travel to infants and children; (3) an actual demonstration of correct restraint-seat anchorage, by the pediatrician in the office; and (4) reminders at the one-month and two-month well-child visits. With these procedures, Reisinger et al. (1981) reported correct usage rates ranging from 38 percent at hospital discharge to 52 percent at 15-month follow-up.

Christophersen & Gyulay (1981) examined the effects of using a single office visit, wherein the positive aspects of restraint-seat usage were emphasized (cf. Christophersen, 1977) and the mother was given a written set of instructions on how to interact with her toddler both when he was riding pleasantly in his restraint seat and when he was attempting to climb out of his restraint seat. This produced striking results with mothers who previously were not using such seats with their toddlers. After the single office visit, correct usage rates increased from zero to 52 percent of the parents in the study, with follow-up data of 75 percent at three months, 62 percent at six months, and 37 percent one full year later.

Christophersen & Sullivan (in press) reported on a crucial variable affecting whether new mothers actually use a restraint seat on the first ride home from the hospital. In the control condition, chosen to represent accurately the typical hospital discharge for a mother and her well newborn (and where the hospital nurse almost never mentioned automobile safety), none of the mothers used a restraint seat on the first ride home. In contrast, in the experimental condition, the hospital staff offered the new mother a loaner restraint seat and actually showed the mother how to place the infant into the restraint correctly, how to carry the infant in the seat to the automobile, and how to fasten the restraint seat correctly on the ride home from the hospital. Sixty-seven percent of the mothers in the experimental group transported their infant in a correctly fastened infant restraint seat. These later studies clearly indicate a developing technology for impacting child morbidity/mortality by increasing car-seat usage.

Burns

Although burns represent the second greatest threat to children, the topic of prevention of burns to children has received relatively little attention in the pediatric literature. In one of the only papers dealing with attempts to get parents to purchase and install smoke detectors, Reisinger, Miller, Blatter, Wucher, & Williams (in press) demonstrated that the pediatrician could be very successful in altering parents' behavior with regard to smoke detectors. The experimental group was given a pamphlet on the hazards of home fires to read while waiting to see the pediatrician. During the office visit, the pediatrician discussed the issues that had been covered in the pamphlet. Smoke detectors were sold at cost in the office to parents in the experimental group. Forty-seven percent of the parents who did not already have a smoke detector purchased one in the pediatrician's office, with 73 percent of these detectors correctly installed when a comprehensive home-safety inspection was carried out four to six weeks later.

Infections

The third most frequent cause of death in children is infectious illness. Chapter 8 of this book, on compliance, specifically addresses the issue of compliance with treatment regimens. Because the pediatrician regularly makes suggestions to parents and/or writes prescriptions that require parental compliance, this is a major area of concern in reducing mortality among children.

Behavior Problems

A third method of prioritizing issues to be addressed by behavioral pediatrics relates to the office management of behavior problems. One obvious way to determine the province of the pediatrician with regard to behavior problems is to examine what kinds of problems children most commonly exhibit or the kinds of problems for which parents commonly solicit advice from the pediatrician.

Richman, Stevenson, & Graham (1975) surveyed over 700 families in a London borough to ascertain the types of problems encountered with three-year-old girls and boys. Table 1.1 is an adaptation of their data. As the table shows, the most common behavior problems were in such areas as bed wetting, toilet training, and sleep problems. These data are very similar to those presented by Reisinger & Bires (1980), who found that feeding problems were the topic discussed most frequently regarding children from birth to two years old, with growth and development of greatest concern regarding two- to four-year-olds.

Table 1.1
Ranked Behavior Problems in Three-Year-Old Boys and Girls

Boys	Girls
Night wetting	Night wetting
Day wetting (1 time per wk.)	Poor appetite
Soiling (1 time per wk.)	Fears
Poor appetite	Waking at night (3 times per wk.)
Overactivity	Sleeping with parents
Difficulty going to bed	Day wetting (1 time per wk.)
Waking at night (3 times per wk.)	Faddy eater
Difficulty controlling	Relations with sibs
Faddy eater	Overactivity
Sleeping with parents	Difficulty going to bed
Relations with sibs	Attention seeking

Source: Adapted from Richman, Stevenson, & Graham (1975).

Probably the most important point to be made from these two surveys is that young children naturally exhibit, and parents freely discuss with their pediatrician, problems that are not usually associated with psychopathology. That is, the problems typically seen by the pediatrician probably are not appropriate for referral to a mental health professional. There are three basic reasons for making this assumption. The first is that the problems are so common that the mental health system probably would be inundated if pediatricians started referring all of the sleeping, eating, and toilet-training problems detected in the normal course of pediatric practice. The second is that there is a serious question as to whether the parents would go to a mental health professional and pay the price for consultation for problems that they did not consider serious and problems that most of their family and friends report having seen before and described as "normal." The third and perhaps most important reason is that most mental health professionals are not trained to deal with common problems of growth and development in the absence of individual or family pathology. Because the pediatrician is the only professional routinely offering well-child care, a much more efficient use of time would be to train the pediatrician how to triage behavior problems and then how to manage the typical behavior problems that are not appropriate for referral.

The issue of triaging behavior problems has not really been addressed in the literature and certainly would merit further investigation. Before pediatricians can decide on the appropriate management of a behavior problem, however, they must be trained to ascertain that it exists in the first place. Starfield & Borkowf (1969) conducted a study wherein they arranged to have mothers of young children interviewed prior to a regularly scheduled appointment with the child's pediatrician. The purpose of this pre-interview was to ascertain the presence of somatic (referring to bodily functions) and behavioral concerns. The pediatricians were able to recognize 78 percent of the mothers' somatic concerns but only 41 percent of the mothers' concerns regarding their child's behavior. In fact, in a typical well-child visit, the pediatricians' mean number of statements about behavior was only 1.6 (Bergman et al., 1966).

One obvious explanation for the physician's lack of recognition of behavioral concerns is that the physician probably is not looking for them. That is, if the pediatrician is not trained to recognize common behavior problems then he probably also is not trained to manage them; hence the apparent inability to recognize behavior problems. The Task Force on Pediatric Education, in their 1978 report, stated that biosocial or behavioral pediatrics was identified by the practicing pediatrician as the most underemphasized area of learning during the pediatric residency training. Whereas the practicing general pediatricians reported spending only 2 percent (on the average) of their time using skills learned in subspecialty areas of pediatrics, fully 65 percent of their time in training was devoted to subspecialty training (e.g., neonatology or hematology–oncology). Obviously, one reason for this discrepancy in training versus practice is that the type of setting in which the training is done (typically a tertiary care center) is well staffed with subspecialists who require the assistance of pediatric residents to cover the patient load in their practices. Another reason, though, has to do with the fact that general or ambulatory pediatrics has never been given the status of a subspecialty area of training. In many residency training programs, ambulatory training must be gleaned from the time spent in the outpatient clinic. All too often, the little training that a resident receives in management of behavior problems comes at the hands of a child psychiatrist who is well versed in psychopathology but who cannot provide well-child care to normal families. Hence, many of the training programs for pediatricians emphasize the importance of establishing rapport with a family in order to help them recognize and work through their problems. There is little recognition of the fact that the general pediatrician, after years of well-child care and episodic management of acute illness, frequently already has established a good working relationship with the parents. This is probably the reason why The Task Force on Pediatric Education (1978) recommends that behavioral pediatrics should be taught by the general or ambulatory pediatrician who practices general pediatrics.

Early Detection of Behavior Problems

Christophersen & Rapoff (1979) specifically addressed the issue of how the pediatrician might arrive easily, within the confines of a well-child visit, at a determination that minor behavior problems exist. Under the auspices of "early detection," that is, deciphering clues that the parents are troubled by their child's behavior before they mention it to the pediatrician, they suggest using a standard set of questions which, in principle, parallels the question asking that is a large part of the work-up for certain organic problems, such as otitis media (an ear infection). For example, with otitis, the pediatrician asks the parents if the child has been rubbing his ear, if he has been running a fever, and if his sleeping patterns have been disrupted. If the answers to these questions are affirmative, then the pediatrician uses her otoscope to assist in arriving at a clinical diagnosis of otitis. Obviously, the pediatrician's training includes substantial experience with otitis, including the method of choice for the management of the same—in all likelihood the prescription of an antibiotic.

During a well-child visit for a three year old, the pediatrician can inquire, in a similar straightforward fashion, about what time the child arises in the morning, who awakens her, who dresses her and how long it takes, and when she leaves the house. The answers to these questions can lead the pediatrician to conclude that the parents are experiencing difficulties in getting their three year old dressed in the morning and off to preschool on time. If the pediatrician ascertains that the child is displaying dressing problems (which rarely are associated with pathology in a three year old), then the parents must be provided with a management protocol. The protocol must include several important characteristics: (1) it must be relatively easy to explain, (2) it must not take an inordinate amount of time to explain, (3) it must be standardized such that it can be printed in the form of an instruction sheet for the parents, and (4) it must list some of the possible side-effects of the procedures with some idea of their severity and duration (cf. Drabman & Jarvie, 1977).

Christophesen & Rapoff (1979) include suggested written protocols for such common problem areas as crying at bedtime, getting out of bed, dressing, mealtime, behavior in public places, noncompliance, and guidelines for parents who use a child-restraint seat. Regarding this last topic, the study by Christophersen & Gyulay (1981) examines the use of such a handout and shows very satisfactory results.

Before the pediatrician recommends a simple management protocol, there are several preconditions that must be met (though they usually already have been met as part of well-child care):

1. Relevant organicity must be ruled out by an appropriate physical examination and whatever back-up laboratory work might be indicated.
2. Significant family psychopathology must be ruled out.
3. Significant marital discord, aside from discord that stems from the presenting behavior problem, must be identified.
4. Provision for either telephone follow-up or a return to the office must be included.
5. The pediatrician must have enough of a working knowledge of normal child development to ascertain that this child's behavior is out of the normal range.

Moderate-to-Severe Behavior Problems

As has been discussed previously, child psychiatrists and clinical child psychologists are trained in the evaluation of and intervention procedures used with children who are experiencing moderate-to-severe behavior problems. The pediatrician who is interested in providing care for these types of problems has several options available. One would be to return to residency training in child psychiatry. A second would be to enroll in a graduate-level program in child development or child psychology that has an emphasis on intervention with young children. The third would be to attend continuing education workshops at local, regional, or national meetings that emphasize the management of a particular problem area.

Obviously, a pediatrician who sees between 25 and 50 patients each day is not in a position to, and usually is not interested in, managing moderate-to-severe behavioral problems. The best course to take, in this case, is to identify whatever mental health services are available in the area of the patient's residence and arrange for a referral to that agency/practitioner. In connection with such a referral, it is reasonable for the pediatrician to expect the practitioner who manages the referral to follow up the referral with a letter or a call wherein the uncovered problems are detailed (thus aiding the referring pediatrician in that it confirms or repudiates the reason for referral), how long the problems will take to be resolved, and what will be done and by whom.

Concluding Remarks

The relatively narrow definition of the scope of the practicing pediatrician as described in this chapter was not chosen arbitrarily by the author; rather, it reflects an exhaustive search of the literature in an effort to describe as accurately as possible the constraints under which the pediatrician operates [see Barnard & Christophersen (in press) for a thorough review of this literature]. That the pediatrician has little time to devote to each patient is partly a function of learning to streamline office practice and partly a function of the clinical acumen derived from years of practice that allows generally accurate diagnoses to be made on the basis of clinical judgment. If the pediatrician is to integrate much in the way of behavioral pediatrics into practice, several suggestions for future directions in this field seem warranted:

1. Fast, accurate screening tools must be developed.
2. Research and training efforts must be directed at the early detection of behavior problems.
3. Standardized intervention protocols must be developed.
4. A triaging system must be developed to aid the pediatrician in decisions on how to manage/refer a particular behavior problem.

Ideally, as pediatricians begin to incorporate behavioral pediatrics into their practice, individual problems can be identified (e.g., encopresis) that can be managed by pediatricians, leaving the mental health practitioner with more time to handle the moderate-to-severe problems that pediatricians identify but have neither the time nor the training to manage.

Although several authors have suggested that general pediatricians can be trained to manage such difficult problem areas as incest and adolescent suicide (e.g., Friedman, 1975), there is virtually no support for such a position in the literature on ambulatory pediatrics. The pediatrician's time can be spent much more effectively by concentrating on well-child care, including the reduction of morbidity and mortality and the detection and management of commonly encountered behavior problems.

References

Barnard, J. D., & Christophersen, E. R. The management of childhood behavior disorders from a pediatric perspective. In C. T. Twentyman, L. H. Epstein, E. B. Blanchard, & J. V. Brady (eds.), *Progress in behavioral medicine*. New York: Springer, in press.

Bergman, A. B., Dassel, S. W., & Wedgwood, R. J. Time–motion study of practicing pediatricians. *Pediatrics*, 1966 38:2, 254–263.

Christophersen, E. R. Children's behavior during automobile rides: Do car seats make a difference? *Pediatrics*, July 1977, *60*, 69–74.

Christophersen, E. R., & Gyulay, J. Parental compliance with car seat usage: A positive approach with long-term follow-up. *Journal of Pediatric Psychology*, 1981, 6:3, 301–312.

Christophersen, E. R., & Rapoff, M. A. Behavioral problems in children. In G. M. Scipien, M. U. Barnard, M. A. Chard, J. Howe, & P. J. Phillips (eds.), *Comprehensive pediatric nursing*. 2nd ed. New York: McGraw-Hill, 1979.

Christophersen, E. R., & Sullivan, M. Increasing the protection of newborn infants in cars. *Pediatrics*, in press.

Drabman, R. S., & Jarvie G. Counselling parents of children with behavior problems: The use of extinction and time-out technique. *Pediatrics*, 1977, 59:1, 78–85.

Friedman, S. B. Foreword to Symposium on behavioral pediatrics. *The Pediatric Clinics of North America*, 1975, 22:3. 515–516.

Leake, H. C., Barnard, J. D., & Christophersen, E. R. Evaluation of pediatric resident performance during the well-child visit. *Journal of Medical Education*, April 1978, 53, 361–363.

McConnochie, K. Use of information from the data base. In S. B. Friedman & R. A. Hoekelman (eds.), *Behavioral pediatrics: Psychosocial aspects of child health care*. New York: McGraw-Hill, 1980.

Pless, I. B. Accident prevention and health education: Back to the drawing board? *Pediatrics*, 1978, 62:3, 431–435.

Reisinger, K. S., & Bires, J. A. Anticipatory guidance in pediatric practice. *Pediatrics*, 1980, 66:6, 889–892.

Reisinger, K. S., Miller, R. E., Blatter, M. M., Wucher, F. P., & Williams, A. F. The effect of pediatricians' counseling on the importance of smoke detectors upon subsequent detector installation. *American Journal of Diseases in Children*, in press.

Reisinger, K. S., Williams, A. F., Wells, J. K., John, C. E., Roberts, T. R., & Podgainy, H. J. Effect of pediatricians' counseling on infant restraint use. *Pediatrics*, 1981, 67:2, 201–206.

Richman, N., Stevenson, J. E., & Graham, P. J. Prevalence of behavior problems in 3-year-old children: An epidemiological study in a London borough. *Journal of Child Psychology and Psychiatry*, 1975, 16:4, 277–287.

Starfield, B. Health care delivery system: Organization, control, costs, and effectiveness. In S. B. Friedman & R. A. Hoekelman (eds.), *Behavioral pediatrics: Psychosocial aspects of child health care*. New York: McGraw-Hill, 1980.

Starfield, B., & Borkowf, S. Physicians' recognition of complaints made by parents about their children's health. *Pediatrics*, 1969, 43:2, 168–172.

The Task Force on Pediatric Education. *The future of pediatric education*. Evanston, Ill.: The Task Force on Pediatric Education, 1978.

CHAPTER 2

Recurrent Abdominal Pain Syndrome: How Appropriate Are Our Basic Clinical Assumptions?

Ronald G. Barr, MDCM, FRCP(C)
Michael Feuerstein, Ph.D.

Introduction

Recurrent abdominal pain (RAP) syndrome in children usually refers to a symptom complex in which the paroxysmal occurrence of unexplained episodes of abdominal pain, over a prolonged period of time, are the cardinal feature. Because children with this syndrome typically are well and act normally between pain episodes, the meaning of the symptom is an enigma to the children themselves, their parents, and the physicians or other therapists to whom they may present for help. While little is known about what the children and their parents take the symptom to mean, clinical practice and the available literature suggest that physicians make the following two assumptions: (1) the cause of the syndrome must be either "organic" or "psychogenic," and (2) the presence of the symptom (pain) indicates the presence of disease, whether organic or psychogenic.

To the extent that these assumptions are brought to bear on the clinical encounter involving the child with RAP, the family, and the physician, they represent a model by which the complaint is given meaning and physicians guide their actions diagnostically and therapeutically. The RAP

The authors would like to acknowledge Dr. Melvin Levine and Dr. Craig Liden, Children's Hospital Medical Center, Boston, for their assistance in compiling the behavioral data; and Mrs. Margaret Campeau for excellent secretarial assistance.

syndrome will be examined to see how this model is applied and whether there are some limitations of the model to be borne in mind when applying it in the clinical setting. The results suggest that our present clinical assumptions should be modified. Since the complaint of recurrent abdominal pain in childhood often is considered a paradigmatic example of a "psychosomatic" complaint, these findings may have implications for our approach to other clinical problems in behavioral medicine.

Characteristics of the Recurrent Abdominal Pain Syndrome

All available research has accepted Apley's[1] operational definition (1975) limiting the syndrome to school-aged children whose pain is 1) paroxysmal in nature; 2) occurs frequently over an extended time period, greater than three episodes over three months or more; and 3) is severe enough to result in a change in activity. The complaint is common, having a prevalance of 10 to 15 percent in school-aged children (Apley, 1975; Oster, 1972; Parcel, Nader, and Meyer, 1977). "Paroxysmal" pain refers to the fact that the appearance of the pain is unpredictable and unexpected and that it also is self-limited, usually lasting less than one hour (Apley, 1975; Roy, Silverman, & Cozzetto, 1975). As mentioned, the child will be well and functioning as usual following the demise of the pain episode. The pain is difficult to describe, other than by its location, which is most commonly periumbilical. Descriptions of the pain elsewhere in the abdomen often are considered a sign that the pain is more likely "organic" in origin (Apley, 1975). The clinical description usually includes a number of associated complaints, which may or may not be present, such as nausea, vomiting, pallor, perspiration, headache, and limb pains (Apley, 1975; Liebman, 1978; Roy et al., 1975; Stone & Barbero, 1970). Complaints implicating organic disease, such as fever, jaundice, bloody stools, pain on urination, urgency, or weight loss seldom are elicited. There are probably more than 100 conditions that may present as unexplained abdominal pain (Bain, 1974); however, the presently available data suggest that the likelihood of finding a disease process accounting for the symptom is less than 10 percent in children hospitalized for the complaint (Apley, 1975), and considerably less in most outpatient series (e.g., Liebman, 1978). It has been reported that two to six percent of patients develop subsequent organic disease (Christensen & Mortensen, 1975; Stickler & Murphy, 1979), but persistence of

---

[1]The debt of the authors to Dr. Apley's important contributions will become more evident during the chapter. In addition, however, there is hardly an article in the literature that does not refer to his work, usually in the first paragraph.

the complaint occurs in over one-third of the patients and "nervous" symptomatology in another third (Apley & Hale, 1973; Christensen & Mortensen, 1975; Stickler & Murphy, 1979). The most common treatment modality consists of child or family counseling directed at possible psychosocial or emotional stresses or "reassurance." No controlled clinical trials of treatment have been reported, with the possible exception of earlier symptom resolution in some patients (Apley & Hale, 1973) and a single case report of symptom resolution by use of "time-out" periods (Miller & Kratchowill, 1979).

This brief review describes the typical medical presentation of the child with RAP and may be referred to as the simple RAP syndrome. Of equal importance, but seldom described, are the secondary consequences to the child with RAP syndrome when interacting with his family, peers, social institutions (e.g., school), and the medical care system. These secondary consequences of the extended RAP syndrome appear to follow from the specific diagnostic dilemma facing physicians. On the one hand, the possibility of missing an occult disease process may stimulate extensive and often invasive investigations. In one clinical series, for example, over 950 tests were conducted in 119 patients, including 185 contrast radiologic studies, 19 esophagoscopies, and 22 electroencephalograms, all with negative results (Liebman, 1978). In a large pediatric hospital there were no positive findings in 100 consecutive upper-gastrointestinal series and 700 consecutive barium enema examinations for the symptom of nonspecific abdominal pain (Cumming, 1979). Finally, in a controlled series of unreferred school children, Apley (1975) reported an appendectomy rate of 5 percent in children with pain compared to 0.3 percent in those without. On the other hand, the relatively infrequent finding of organic disease, especially in ambulatory patients, results in many physicians doing little investigation for organic disease and assuming a psychogenic etiology. However, recent studies suggest that, with more sensitive and appropriate diagnostic assessments, an assumption of psychogenic etiology may be inappropriate and misleading in some patients (Barr, Levine, & Watkins, 1979; Goldstein, deCholnoky, Leventhal, & Emans, 1979). In sum, part of the extended RAP syndrome includes inappropriate diagnostic workups, inaccurate labeling, and, as a result, significantly increased morbidity.

Psychogenic Recurrent Abdominal Pain

In light of the consequences of the extended RAP syndrome, it is of considerable importance that the possible role of "psychogenicity" in the etiology of RAP be considered carefully, since, almost without exception, children who suffer from nonorganic recurrent abdominal pain are considered to have psychogenic pain accounting for the symptom. While the exact meaning of the term *psychogenic* may be outmoded (Engel, 1977) and, according to many authors, far from clear, a common concept in most descriptions is that stressful, emotional, or psychosocial factors have some role in the production of the syndrome. In order to understand their role better, it will be useful to distinguish among the factors that predispose individuals to RAP syndrome, those that exacerbate or precipitate a pain episode, and those that maintain the syndrome. While psychogenicity would seem to imply that the aforementioned factors predispose a child to RAP syndrome, specific etiologic evidence of their role is lacking, since there are no prospective studies identifying psychosocial or emotional stress as risk factors. Therefore, the focus of this discussion will be placed on psychogenicity as an exacerbating or maintaining factor.

In his landmark monograph, *The Child with Abdominal Pains* (Apley, 1975), the late John Apley paid considerable attention to the role that stress or emotional disturbance might play in RAP syndrome. It is worth considering his work carefully, not only because he contributed important empirical data previously missing, but also because of his enormous influence on all of the subsequent literature on the subject. He observed that "there had previously been no considerable body of evidence to suggest that there is an increased frequency of abdominal pain in children at times when emotional disturbances occur or that such disturbances precede the onset of attacks of pain. The data from the present studies have filled some of the gaps and compelled me to modify my views" (p. 90). Reviewing the studies, he observed that "from all the evidence it appears justifiable to conclude that, in a large proportion of children with recurrent abdominal pain, the criteria of a stress disorder are fulfilled" (p. 93). The qualifiers in Dr. Apley's conclusions are important, both to acknowledge their tentativeness and to prevent oversimplistic interpretations of his findings. As mentioned, his conclusions often have been taken in the literature and in practice to mean that RAP is either organic or psychogenic, an interpretation that goes beyond both his data and his own conclusions. Nevertheless, this dualistic interpretation has much appeal and apparent validity in the clinical setting, and it may be worth examining why this is so. Our review will suggest that the role of stress in RAP is still far from clear and that other subgroups of patients must not be overlooked in the process.

To structure the discussion we will adopt Apley's "elementary criteria" to justify a diagnosis of emotional or "stress" disorder, namely: (1) there should be reasonably adequate negative evidence to eliminate an organic cause; (2) there should be positive evidence that there is an emotional disturbance and that the disorder may be related in time with periods of increased stress; and (3) the disorder should respond to measures directed at the relief of emotional tension (Apley, 1975).

Elimination of Organic Causes

Concerning the first criterion, there is little debate that, for most children with RAP, an organic cause is seldom found. In those studies reporting higher prevalence of organic causes (e.g., Rahman, Singh, Agarwal, & Srivastava, 1978; Goldstein et al., 1979), the populations appeared to be highly select or not comparable to North American or British practices. Two important qualifiers should be noted, however. The first is Apley's warning (1975) that, in many cases, organic anomalies may be detected that are unrelated to the pain complaint. Claims for organic causes hardly can be acceptable in the absence of appropriate longitudinal follow-up in such patients. The second qualifier is that the phrase *organic cause* is ambivalent. It may refer either to organ disease producing the pain symptom or to normal physiological functioning resulting in pain symptoms. As discussed later, overlooking this semantic distinction probably contributes to inappropriately labeling the symptom psychogenic.

Evidence of Emotional Causes

The second criterion, that there should be positive evidence of emotional disturbance and that the disorder should be related in time with periods of increased stress, is more problematic. As evidence for emotional disturbance, Apley & Naish (1958) reported their findings in unselected school children with appropriate controls with regard to intelligence, emotional disturbances, and personality. Although there were no differences in intelligence between the groups, undue fears, nocturnal enuresis, sleep disorders, and appetite difficulties were reported significantly more often in children with RAP than controls. It was concluded that "many more children with pains tended to be highly-strung, fussy, excitable, anxious, timid and apprehensive" (p. 168). Unfortunately, although these data were collected using a semistructured interview including an unspecified number of comparisons, only the summary data were reported.

In the clinical setting, the impression of a higher prevalence of behavioral and emotional disturbance is likely to be confirmed. Use of a standard questionnaire in a general ambulatory clinic of a large pediatric hospital gave us the opportunity to examine how frequently such behaviors were reported in a clinical population. Data from a comparison group in a nearby low- and middle-income working-class community also were collected as part of a normative study on neurodevelopmental function. Children with learning disabilities and known psychiatric or physically handicapping conditions were excluded. Since these data were collected for different purposes, they cannot be considered a control group, which would have required stricter matching procedures. Nevertheless, available comparisons showed that there were no statistically significant differences between the groups as to age, sex, or number of siblings in the families.

Parents were asked to respond to 54 statements (see Table 2.1) concerning the behavior of the children (e.g., "He/she cries easily") by checking one of these replies: "definitely applies," "applies somewhat," "does not apply," or "cannot say." For purposes of this analysis, the first two responses are coded as "yes," the last two as "no." Affirmative responses of the comparison-group parents to the statement, "He/she has stomachaches often" ($n = 17$) permitted the subgroups (comparison, non-pain; comparison, pain) to be considered separately. Probability levels are derived from χ^2 analyses.

Simple inspection of the overall results suggested that, for the physician in the clinical setting, it would be easy to find "positive" evidence of behavioral problems in children presenting with RAP. Indeed, consistent with Apley's findings suggesting a particular personality profile, the pattern of findings that were statistically significant seemed to cluster around items that fit the description of the children with RAP as "anxious, timid,

Table 2.1

Behavioral Problems in Clinical Recurrent Abdominal Pain and Unreferred Comparison Groups (percentage affirmative responses)

	Group				
	Clinical		Comparison		
Item	RAP ($n = 80$)	Sig.[1]	Non-pain ($n = 82$)	Sig.[2]	Pain ($n = 17$)
1. Constant motion	59		49		59
2. Overactive mind	47		31		41
3. Starts, does not finish	56		48		41
4. Trouble falling asleep	49	***	20		41
5. Distracts easily	51		26		38
6. Keeps changing games	39		22		29
7. Can't keep hands to self	18		21		12
8. Always wants things	45		23		23
9. Moody	54		48		41
10. Bad temper	42		37		29

11. Cries easily	64	*	46		63
12. Worrier	62	*	41	*	71
13. Bad dreams	39	*	21		33
14. Often sad	38	**	17		18
15. Often very quiet	36		32		41
16. Whines often	32		21		24
17. Many fears	40	**	17		19
18. Often tired	49	***	12		24
19. Stutters/stammers	10		4		6
20. Wets bed/pants	7		12		6
21. Headaches	57	***	9	***	41
22. Overeats	31	**	11		18
23. Bites nails	31		17		24
24. Sucks thumb/objects	18		20		0
25. Nervous twitches	12		4		0
26. Feels ill often	66	***	5	**	30
27. Too neat/orderly	32	**	12		18
28. Too concerned with cleanliness	32	**	7		6
29. Tells lies	28		28		19
30. Steals at home	1		5		0
31. Plays with matches	3		4		0
32. Smokes cigarettes	0		1		0
33. Bullies children	12		12		18
34. Uses foul language	11		7		12
35. Destroys objects home	4		7		0
36. Destroys objects away	3		0		0
37. Fearless	31		20		31
38. Cheats in games	26		19		33
39. Skips school	4		0		0
40. Trouble w/ neighbors	9		1		0
41. Cruel to animals	1		0		0
42. Loner	26		25		29
43. No real friends	15		5		6
44. Loses friends easily	11		5		6
45. Mostly younger friends	23		11		13
46. Mostly older friends	27		19		19
47. Mostly opposite sex friends	19	*	5		0
48. No best friend	19		15		12
49. Prefers adult friends	18	*	5		12
50. Gets picked on	37	*	19		35
51. Jealous easily	41	*	25		41
52. Not liked by other children	14		9		6
53. Slow to make friends	19		21		30

[1]Statistical significance by χ^2 analysis of clinical RAP vs. comparison group without abdominal pain (non-pain).
[2]Statistical significance by χ^2 analysis of comparison group without abdominal pain (non-pain) vs. comparison group with abdominal pain (pain).
*$p<0.05$
**$p<0.01$
***$p<0.001$

and apprehensive" (particularly items 11, 12, and 14) and as having "undue fears" (item 17) and "sleep disorders" (items 4, 13, and 18). In addition, these items tended to be more common in unreferred children with pain, although the smaller number in this group may have prevented them from being statistically significant, with the exception of item 12. The increased prevalence of enuresis (item 20) did not appear to be confirmed in this data. Certainly, there was no suggestion that these children "acted out" more than the comparison group (items 29 through 41).

This apparent confirmation may not be as strong as it seems for a number of reasons. First, the questionnaire for the referred group of children with RAP was completed as part of a clinical diagnostic evaluation; hence, parents may have been more sensitized to their childrens' problems in this setting, producing a higher rate of positive responses. Second, for both Apley's data and ours, there is no way of knowing whether these behavioral characterstics were the causes or the effects of being a child with RAP. Third, since similar behavior characterstics also were fairly common in the comparison group, averaging 17 percent for the items that were statistically significantly different, the clinician faced with evaluating an individual child had a difficult time distinguishing whether the presence of these characteristics was associated with, or just incidental to, the pain complaint. Finally, because of the large number of comparisons, one would expect that two to three comparisons would reach statistical significance by chance, and two of the most significant positive associations (item 21 and 26) describe characteristics of the syndrome itself. Thus, while the pattern of behaviors in the referred population appeared to be fairly consistent with that described in Apley's nonreferred population, and while it also is highly likely that behavioral or emotional problems in general will be reported by parents of patients presenting with RAP, the strength of this particular association and its clinical significance in any particular case may be less than it appeared on the surface. A properly controlled study including a "positive" control group of hospital visitors with other complaints is necessary to conclude that children with RAP have a personality profile specific to the syndrome.

Perhaps the strongest cautionary argument against understanding all the children with nonorganic RAP as psychogenic on the basis of behavioral data is Apley's own findings (1975) that 51 percent of the children with RAP were classified as "normal, average, good." He also noted that, of 92 hospitalized children without organic disorder, there was "an outstandingly interesting group of thirteen children" with negative evidence of emotional disturbance and another 12 children (27 percent) with insufficient evidence. Consequently, while emotional disturbance may well be operative at some level in an important subgroup of children, not all nonorganic RAP can reasonably be considered psychogenic.

Clinical reports implicating "stress" in the etiology of RAP syndrome usually describe experiences that may act as "trigger" events to exacerbate the pain symptoms. Thus, many authors (Apley, 1975; Liebman, 1978; Green, 1967; Heinild, Malner, Roelsgaard, & Worning, 1959; Stone, 1970; Roy et al., 1975; Poznanski, 1976; Hughes & Zimin, 1978) listed school entrance, family quarrels and separations, marital distress, changes in environment, and so on as being particularly prevalent in the lives of children with RAP. Most persuasive in this regard was the experience reported by Apley (1975) in which specific case histories were provided and the essential temporal relation between triggering event and the pain experience was described. Apley claimed that precipitating factors for the attacks of pain were elicited in one-third of children as determined by a semistructured interview. He stated further that a clear relationship between stress and the first pain attack was obtained in "a few" children, whereas a relationship between recurrent attacks and stress was evident in "many" children. Green (1967) cautioned, however, that, while such stressors appear to be etiologically relevant, a direct relationship between the symptom and the stressful situation was uncommon. Most authors simply reported a high prevalence of presumably stressful events elicited during history taking, with no mention of the temporal proximity or sequential relationship to the target symptoms. While the apparent unanimity on the part of so many authors would seem to substantiate the hypothesis, no studies have provided controlled data on this point. In addition, the simple presence of a life event does not mean that it is stressful, and equal attention seldom was paid to whether these children showed positive evidence of having coped with these presumably stressful life events. In summary, available data are at present inadequate to judge whether children with RAP experience more stress episodes than controls. Neither is there data to determine whether their response to the same stress is different from that found in non-RAP controls.

Another important possible flaw in these studies concerns the bias of ascertainment that may result from the documented fact that stress episodes have been shown to increase the likelihood that a child will be seen by a physician, regardless of whether the symptom is stress related or not (Roghmann & Haggerty, 1973). In addition, the frequency of reported stress episodes (three to four per month, each lasting two to three days) makes it difficult to distinguish incidental from etiologic stress events at least in the clinical context (Roghmann & Haggerty, 1973). Green (1967) noted that the abdominal pain attack may only be the occasion for bringing other family problems to light for help from a health care professional.

The other sense in which the term psychogenic is used is to denote factors that maintain the complaint of abdominal pain. However, evidence pertaining to factors that maintain stress-related abdominal pain symptoms is less plentiful than evidence that stress exacerbates abdominal pain symptoms. Conceptualizations of how the pain symptom may be maintained usually fall into two categories. First, a specific target organ (e.g., intestine) becomes specifically subject to manifesting the effects of stress through contingent reinforcement (Blendis, Hill, & Merskey, 1978), either by increased attention or by the reestablishment of a particular balance of interpersonal or intrafamilial relationships (Apley, 1975; Craig, 1978). Second, the "malingering" hypothesis assumes that abdominal pain is not actually felt but that the verbal complaint behavior acts as an effective mechanism for avoidance of unwanted experiences (Apley, 1975; Poznanski, 1976). In both cases, the environment is regarded as playing a major role in the maintenance of the complaint through reinforcement of the pain behavior or through a modeling process. Thus, with regard to reinforcement, there are many anecdotal observations describing parents of children with RAP as overprotective (Apley, 1975), demonstrating "contagious circular anxiety" (Stone, 1970), having "a compulsion to find something wrong with (their) child" (Green, 1967) or "anxious—sometimes to the point of panic" (Hughes, 1978), any of which could provide the setting for such reinforcement. Once again, however, control data are lacking. Similarly, the possibility of pain modeling was suggested by findings of an increased prevalence of abdominal pain complaints in parents and siblings of children who complained of pain, when compared to controls (Apley, 1975; Oster, 1972; Stone, 1970). While such a correlation was consistent with either a modeling hypothesis or a constitutional predisposition, Christensen & Mortensen (1975) reported that abdominal pain occurred no more frequently among children of parents who were complaining of pain at the time of investigation than among children whose parents were without such symptoms. This latter finding is more consistent with the modeling hypothesis.

Responsiveness to Psychotherapy

In discussing evidence in favor of Apley's third criterion, that the symptom be responsive to measures directed at relief of emotional tension, Apley (1975) compared results in two series of cases that were followed up eight to 14 years later. An earlier series of 30 patients was "untreated," and the later series was "treated." Treatment was described as "informal psychotherapy," ranging from simple reassurance that organic disease had been excluded to sympathetic listening and advice on changing environmental factors that might contribute to tension. Primarily, the results indicated that there were no differences in the number of children (1) free from abdominal symptoms; (2) free from abdominal symptoms but with other complaints, pains, or nervous symptoms, or (3) with continuing abdominal symptoms (approximately one-third in each group). However, the pains ceased "promptly" in 75 percent of treated cases as compared with 20 percent of untreated cases, and the total number of other symptoms was somewhat less in the treated group (24 symptoms in 21 patients) than in the untreated group (41 symptoms in 21 patients). Apley also made two other important clinical observations. The first was the uncontrolled observation that, in the treated series, the pains were less severe and less frequent in nine of the 11 patients in whom stomach pains persisted. The second was that treatment "seemed also to increase the patient's adaptability and make it more likely that he could live a normal life" (p. 62). Evidence for this latter statement was that work and activity were restricted in only two patients.

As Apley himself suggested, much work could be done profitably on devising more sophisticated approaches to informal psychotherapy. In addition, the suggestion that informal psychotherapy of whatever sort permits better adaptability on the part of the patient points out another legitimate benefit. However, the fact that an equal number of patients continued to have pain in both groups would be consistent with the suggestion that, for a significant subgroup of these patients, other factors not as responsive to informal psychotherapy are likely to be operative. Indeed, a more parsimonious explanation of these results might be that informal counseling reduced the secondary anxiety resulting from being a child with abdominal pain, rather than removing the anxiety that may have caused the pain. While this is certainly a legitimate clinical objective, it does not support the claim that all nonorganic abdominal pain is psychogenic.

The Assumption of Disease

Let us turn briefly to the second commonly made clinical assumption; namely, that the presence of the symptom (pain) indicates the presence of disease, whether organic or psychogenic. For purposes of this discussion, *disease* will be interpreted rather broadly as "something wrong" or "abnormal." The main point is that our usual clinical model seldom includes a category of normal children who may have the pain symptom for normal reasons. The lack of appropriate recognition of such a possibility and the lack of appropriate diagnostic tools for assessing it may result in more attributions of psychogenicity than are warranted.

Recent studies on the role of lactose intolerance in recurrent abdominal pain raises the possibility that pain episodes may occur as a result of the interaction between a normal constitutional factor (low levels of small-intestine lactose activity during school age) and a normal environmental factor (ingestion of lactose). Despite the knowledge that incomplete lactose absorption could produce the symptoms of abdominal pain, diarrhea, bloating, and gas, little information was available on whether this mechanism might account for a subgroup of children with RAP. Using the noninvasive lactose breath hydrogen test to screen for ability to absorb lactose (Barr, Watkins, & Perman, 1981), we found that 20 percent of a mixed Caucasian population with RAP met the criteria for lactose malabsorption that could account for their symptoms (Barr, Levine, & Watkins, 1979). Similar findings were reported in a study by Liebman (1979), which included a control group of clinic visitors without abdominal pain who were tested for lactose malabsorption. Of some interest was the additional finding that the clinical presentation in terms of pain frequency, milk ingestion, and presence of diarrhea did not distinguish the subgroup of lactose-intolerant children with RAP from the others (Barr et al., 1979). Nor would the usual tests for organic "disease" detect the normally low lactose levels in this group. These findings raise the possibility that the RAP syndrome may be due in some cases to a nonpathologic mechanism and that such a group might be overlooked easily in an evaluation focusing on organic or emotional disease. The extent of the role of lactose intolerance as a factor in RAP is still uncertain, however, both because the crucially important diet trials were uncontrolled and unblinded in these studies and because the prevalence of incomplete lactose absorption will vary according to the ethnic mix of the populations studied.

Conclusions

It has been suggested that the usual clinical model brought to bear in the clinical interaction with the child with RAP includes the following two assumptions: (1) that the cause of the syndrome must be either organic or psychogenic and (2) that the presence of the symptom indicates the presence of disease, whether organic or psychogenic.

With regard to the first assumption, the available evidence is more suggestive that psychogenicity may play a role in an important subgroup of patients with nonorganic RAP. Even in this subgroup, careful attention needs to be paid to how the apparent emotional stresses act, whether they relate to the syndrome as cause or effect, and whether they are incidental to the syndrome but precipitate the clinical visit. Clearly, more well-controlled studies would be helpful in attempting to parse out the role of psychogenicity in this syndrome.

With regard to the second assumption, it seems probable that the presence of the symptom may in some cases not imply disease. In such cases, ruling out organic causes does not exclude normal physiologic processes from being operative, nor does absence of psychopathology imply that "it's all in the head." It appears that both assumptions are poorly supported by the clinical data and need to be reconsidered.

As a first approximation, a revised clinical model should permit a category in which neither organic nor psychogenic etiology is presumed and in which the symptom is not presumed to imply disease. This comparison between the "traditional" model and the proposed model is represented graphically in Figure 2.1. It is perhaps ironic that John Apley, whose work was so important in highlighting the potential role of stress and emotional factors, did not himself accept the "traditional" model. The grouping he recommended included an organic group, a stress group, and a provisional group, the latter to include those that "cannot immediately be placed in either of the above groups" (Apley, 1975, p. 102). Whether he expected that all diagnoses would be subsumed eventually into one or the other of the former groups is unclear, but his provisional group probably would have included those children (51 percent in the unreferred, and 14 percent or more in the hospital group) in whom evidence for organicity or psychogenicity was absent. While the relative sizes and the appropriate

Figure 2.1   Alternative Clinical Models for Recurrent Abdominal Pain Syndrome. The presence of cross-hatching indicates an assumption of "disease" being present. "Dysfunctional" RAP syndrome refers to children in whom appropriate evidence for organicity or psychogenicity is lacking and no assumption of abnormality is made.

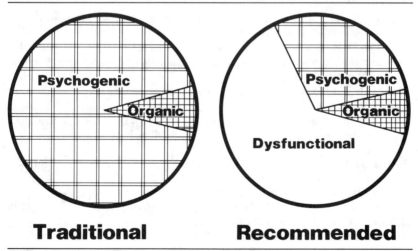

Traditional   **Recommended**

Redrawn and reproduced by permission from Stewart Gable (ed.), *Behavior Problems in Children*. New York: Grune & Stratton, 1981, p. 237.

components of this model are still to be determined, recognition of the limitations of the usual clinical model may be important as an antidote to oversimplistic and inappropriate diagnoses and therapy.

References

Apley, J. *The child with abdominal pain*. London: Blackwell, 1975.

Apley, J., & Hale, B. Children with recurrent abdominal pain. How do they grow up? *Brit. Med. Journal*, 1973, *3*, 7–9.

Apley, J., & Naish, N. Recurrent abdominal pains: A field survey of 1000 school-children. *Archives of Disease in Childhood*, 1958, *33*, 165–170.

Bain, H. W. Chronic vague abdominal pain in children. Pediatric Clinics of North America, 1974, *21*:4, 991–1000.

Barr, R. G., Levine, M. D., & Watkins, J. W. Recurrent abdominal pain of childhood due to lactose intolerance, a prospective study. *New England Journal of Medicine*, June 28, 1979, *300*, 1449–1452.

Barr, R. G., Watkins, J. B., & Perman, J. A. Mucosal function and breath hydrogen excretion: Comparative studies in the clinical evaluation of children with nonspecific abdominal complaints. *Pediatrics*, October 1981, *68*:4, 526–533.

Blendis, L. M., Hill, O. W., & Merskey, H. Abdominal pain and the emotions. *Pain*, 1978, *5*:2, 179–191.

Christensen, M. F., & Mortensen, O. Long-term prognosis in children with recurrent abdominal pain. *Archives of Diseases in Childhood*, 1975, *50*, 110–114.

Craig, K. D. Social modelling influences on pain. In R. A. Sternbach (ed.), *The psychology of pain*. New York: Raven Press, 1978.

Cumming, W. A. Personal communication, 1979.

Engel, G. L. The need for a new medical model: A challenge for biomedicine. *Science*, 1977, *196*, 129–136.

Goldstein, D. P., de Cholnoky, C., Leventhal, J. M., & Emans, S. J. New insights into the old problem of chronic pelvic pain. *Journal of Pediatric Surgery*, 1979, *14*, 675–680.

Green, M. Diagnosis and treatment: Psychogenic recurrent abdominal pain. *Pediatrics*, 1967, *40*, 84–89.

Heinild, S. V., Malner, E., Roelsgaard G., & Worning, B. A psychosomatic approach to recurrent abdominal pain in childhood. *Acta Paediatrica*, 1959, *48*, 361–370.

Hughes, M. L., & Zimin, R. Children with psychogenic abdominal pain and their families. *Clinical Pediatrics*, 1978, *17*, 569–573.

Liebman, W. M. Recurrent abdominal pain in children: A retrospective survey of 119 patients. *Clinical Pediatrics*, 1978, *17*, 149–153.

Liebman, W. M. Recurrent abdominal pain in children: Lactose and sucrose intolerance, a prospective study. *Pediatrics*, 1979, *64*, 43–45.

Miller, A. J., & Kratchowill, T. R. Reduction of frequent stomach-ache complaints by time out. *Behavior Therapy*, 1979, *10*, 211–218.

Oster, J. Recurrent abdominal pain, headache and limb pains in children and adolescents. *Pediatrics*, 1972, *50*, 429–436.

Parcel, G. S., Nader, P. R., & Meyer, M. P. Adolescent health concerns, problems, and patterns of utilization in a triethnic urban population. *Pediatrics*, 1977, *60*, 157–164.

Poznanski, E. O. Children's reaction to pain: a psychiatrist's perspective. *Clinical Pediatrics*, 1976, *15*, 1114–1119.

Rahman, H., Singh, B. B. Agarwal, V. K., & Srivastava, A. K. Abdominal pain in children—a clinical study. *Indian Pediatrics*, 1978, *15*, 583–588.

Roghmann, K. J., & Haggerty, R. J. Daily stress, illness, and use of health services in young families. *Pediatric Research*, 1973, *7*, 520–526.

Roy, C. C., Silverman, A., & Cozzetto, F. J. *Pediatric Clinical Gastroenterology*, St. Louis: C. V. Mosby, 1975.

Stickler, G. B., & Murphy, D. B. Recurrent abdominal pain. *American Journal of Diseases in Children*, 1979, *133*, 486–489.

Stone, R. T., & Barbero, G. J. Recurrent abdominal pain in childhood. *Pediatrics*, 1970, *45*, 732–738.

CHAPTER 3

The Nature of Asthma

A. Barney Alexander, Ph.D.

Incidence and Scope

Bronchial asthma is a disorder that can cause significant disability and disruption of regular life patterns. It is estimated that 8.6 million Americans currently suffer from the disorder (approximately 4 percent of the population) and a total of 14 million people (or 7 percent of the population) either have been in the past or are presently handicapped by asthma (Davis, 1972). Compared to heart disease and cancer, asthma does not have a high mortality rate; however, the disease does account for between 2,000 (Segal, 1976) and 4,000 (Davis, 1972) deaths per year. Additionally, the disabling effects of the disorder on the lives of those who suffer from asthma can be extensive. Asthma is the leading cause of limitation in activity in children under the age of 17, who make up approximately 60 percent of all asthma sufferers (National Center for Health Statistics, 1971). Asthma accounts for almost one quarter of all days lost from school by chronically ill children (Schiffer & Hunt, 1963). During 1968, 134,000 hospitalized patients were diagnosed as having asthma or hay fever and experienced an average yearly hospital stay of 8.3 days, costing approximately $62 million (American Hospital Association, 1971). Furthermore, Davis (1972) suggested that asthma accounted for 5 million days lost from work, 7 million days lost from school, and 27 million patient visits to physicians in one year. The economic costs of asthma were also high. Based on drug industry estimates, Creer (1978) stated that in 1975 patients spent $224.2 million for bronchodilators, $24.7 million for corticosteroids, and $43 million for over-the-counter remedies for asthma. With the additional costs of physician and hospital care, Cooper (1976) estimated that the total cost of asthma in one year, exclusive of mortality, was $1.3 billion.

Description of the Asthmatic

Severe hardships are not uncommon for the childhood asthmatic and his family. These youngsters tend to grow up watching the other children play—from the inside of the living-room window. Poor self-concepts are common, and both academic and social development often suffer greatly due to the amount of time lost from school and the restricted and specialized contacts with both peers and adults, who are overindulgent or lack understanding of the asthmatic's difficulties. Often these children react with shame and embarrassment or extreme demandingness; at home, asthma may become the sole focus around which all family concerns come to revolve. For example, disruption in activities and vacation plans can become common, as well as late-night visits to emergency rooms. Parents sometimes may feel guilty, responsible, and helpless; at other times resentful and angry; on still other occasions, shameful and embarrassed, especially in social or even treatment circumstances where many people still make parents feel that they somehow "caused" the asthma emotionally. Certainly an asthma sufferer can learn to manipulate others with the disorder or use it to excuse poor performance. Since severe physical restrictions are not uncommon, it often is very difficult for the patient to sort out clearly what can be accomplished in the face of asthma. Many maladaptive and inappropriate behavior patterns can develop as patient and family struggle with the ravages of this disorder, and such patterns can cripple family life severely and retard the social and psychological development of the child. Often these undesirable behavior patterns substantially affect the course of the disorder.

Asthma is potentially life threatening, and many patients on occasion have experienced bouts of status asthmaticus that may have brought them close to death. Such experiences often generate enduring anxiety responses that can manifest themselves in fears of death, hospitals, and treatment. Some patients develop conditioned fear responses that can begin at even the first signs of wheezing. The frantic, worried behavior of parents and those treating the patient can exacerbate the young patient's fear. Moods vary with the severity of the symptoms and also in relation to medications taken, from the widespread adrenergic effects (e.g., tremor and concentration difficulties) of the sympathomimetics, to the side-effects of the corticosteroids, which include stunted growth, edema, insomnia, moonface, amenorrhea, delayed sexual development, cataracts, osteoporosis, thromboembolism, learning and memory deficits, and depression. As if these weren't enough, the common cold can become a nightmare of increased asthma symptoms, often of the most serious nature.

The Medical Aspects of Asthma

The Physical Reaction

Bronchial asthma is a syndrome characterized by episodes of obstruction to proper air exchange in the lung, manifested by wheezing respirations, dyspnea, cough, and excessive mucus production. These changes in the bronchi and bronchioles are caused by mucosal edema, hypersecretion of thick mucus, and contraction of bronchial smooth muscle, all of which result in a reduction in the size of the inside diameter of the air-transporting tubes in the lung. In some cases the viscid mucus production results in a complete blocking of the lumen, leading to frank trapping of biologically unusable gas in the part of the lung distal to the plug. An important characteristic of asthma, as opposed to other conditions that may impair the ability of the lung to transport air, is that the symptoms are reversible, either through adequate and appropriate pharmocological means or by virtue of normal remission between attacks. Thus, asthma sufferers may have completely normal pulmonary function in the periods between episodes of asthma, which can be as long as several months or even years.

Types of Asthma

The most widely recognized classification system is that of Rackeman (1928), in which asthma is considered to be either extrinsic (due to allergic reaction), intrinsic (nonallergic, infectious, etc.), or mixed. Most patients fall into the latter category, although extrinsic or intrinsic factors may predominate in any particular case. Nevertheless, for most victims the majority of asthmatic symptoms are related to allergens. While initial sensitization usually requires a very large antigen load, once sensitization has taken place, highly allergic individuals may experience symptoms following even minute exposures. Common asthmogenic allergens include tree, grass, and weed pollens; molds and fungi; animal danders and feathers; house and occupational dusts; some foods; insects (but not their stings); and some chemicals (but not in their role as irritants).

Nonallergic asthmogenic stimuli include aspirin, exercise, airway irritants, certain situations, and infections. Though rather uncommon, aspirin idiosyncrasy can cause dangerously violent symptoms in some asthmatics. Exercise is such a common asthma precipitant that exercise-induced bronchospasm has been suggested as a defining characteristic of asthma. Individual sensitivity varies from mild to severe in specific individuals but manifests a fairly tight relationship to extent of exertion in any particular case. Usually, exercise-induced asthma reverses nonproblematically with rest and appropriate medication. Common airway irritants include certain chemical gases, aerosol propellants, cold air, and cough. Hyperventilation may cause bronchospasm, both by airway irritation and hypocapnia. Other circumstances, such as certain weather conditions and weather changes, can precipitate asthma idiosyncratically in many patients by as yet unknown means. Respiratory infections represent one of the most common asthma precipitants and are the cause of some of the most severe and prolonged episodes, often requiring hospitalization and life-saving therapy. Although it is uncertain whether bacterial infections may provoke asthma, it now is known that viral infections such as colds and influenza are the cause of most infection-induced asthma.

Prognosis

Despite many attempts, precise prognostic data are difficult to obtain. As many as 40 percent of all asthmatics may show substantial or complete remission of symptoms as they grow older, especially during the early teenage years. This intriguing "outgrowing" of asthma, as well as the natural course and ultimate outcome in general, seem to relate, even if inperfectly, to many factors. Certainly the severity of asthma after onset relates positively to the likelihood of persistence of symptoms. Sex differences also exist, with males being afflicted twice as often as females, although this proportion evens out at puberty. Not only are girls less likely to be afflicted than boys, but the latter are slightly less likely to experience a remission of symptoms during adulthood. Poorer prognosis is associated with appearance of symptoms before the age of two or after the age of 25. It also seems to be the case that allergic individuals manifest a greater incidence of more severe and persistent symptoms. In contrast, asthma in children, which seems to be due largely to respiratory infections, suggests a more favorable prognosis. Despite these trends and the clear expectation of partial or complete remission over time for many asthmatic children, the strength of these relationships is such that treatment strategy in individual cases (such as highly conservative therapy) cannot be decided upon by the expectation of ultimate favorable outcome for many sufferers. Also, former symptomatic asthma victims typically manifest lingering evidence of lung hypersensitivity and show a clear tendency to experience symptoms under unfavorable conditions. Finally, one note of optimism can be struck by the fact that irreversible lung damage does not seem to be associated significantly with asthma, whatever its severity or duration.

Etiology

The etiology of asthma remains incompletely understood, but in some instances much has been learned regarding the pathogenesis of asthma symptoms. Of the two broad classes of asthmogenic stimuli—allergic and nonallergic—attention has been focused, understandably, on the former. A substantial proportion of asthma symptoms can be attributed to the antigen–antibody reaction, especially in the less severe asthmatic whose symptoms are largely seasonal. Nevertheless, it is clear that immunologic mechanisms by no means can account for all incidences of asthma. The three most important nonimmunologic pathogenic factors are hyperirritability of the airways, exercise-induced bronchospasm, and infection-caused asthma. The first has been studied extensively and the existence of a vagally mediated irritant reflex that results in bronchial constriction has been demonstrated. The second, exercise-induced asthma, is understood less well but may involve either or both the release of chemical mediators of the kind found in the allergic response (such as histamine, SRS-A, and some prostaglandins) or the previously mentioned irritant reflex through stimulation by insufficiently warmed air during exertion. The third factor, respiratory infections, are not only potent asthma precipitants but tend to be the immediate precursor to the first appearance of asthma for the majority of individuals. The mechanisms involved in infectious asthma are still quite speculative, and, in terms of overall development, the most comprehensive etiologic theory to date is known as the *beta adrenergic blockage* proposed by Szentivanyi (1968). According to this theory, asthmatics manifest a reduced responsivity of the bronchodilatory beta adrenergic receptors in the lung, leaving the lung relatively unprotected from both vagal and humoral constricting factors. Unfortunately, as appealing as this theory may be, the supporting evidence remains highly equivocal.

Genetics

An understanding of the contribution of genetic factors in allergy and asthma disorders has been delayed by the almost complete lack of standardization of definitional, sampling, and assessment criteria. The best twin data to date (Edfors-Lubs, 1971) suggests that familial factors may play a substantially less prominent role than was assumed previously. In this study, a concordance rate in monozygotic twins was only 19 percent for asthma and 25 percent for all allergic disorders. Both of these figures were only marginally higher than the corresponding figure for dizygotic twins. Further, the results indicated only a 1-in-3 chance that a child would develop allergies when both parents were atopic and showed that the majority of allergic children were born into families in which neither parent or only one parent manifested atopy.

Diagnosis

Clinically, the diagnosis of asthma is based largely upon the patient's history, certain laboratory tests, and, to a lesser extent, characteristic physical findings. A careful and complete history is of crucial importance.

Typically, episodic dyspnea, chest tightness, and wheezing or cough are reported. Extensive probing for precipitants of attacks usually will reveal whether the asthma manifests a substantial allergic (extrinsic) component or is largely infectious (intrinsic). Complete information regarding the physical environment—including places frequented away from home, reactions to exercise, and the periodicity of attacks, nocturnal symptoms, and so on—is essential to both the diagnosis and subsequent treatment planning. A family history of allergy or asthma is not uncommon, though a negative family history by no means precludes a diagnosis of asthma or even allergy.

Physical examination findings depend to a great extent upon the condition of the patient at the time. It must be remembered that one of the cardinal characteristics of asthma is its periodicity. As a consequence the patient may exhibit perfectly normal air exchange during periods between episodes. In some cases, especially in children, patients with histories of chronic asthma may exhibit characteristic barrel-chest deformities due to chronic hyperinflation. The eyes, ears, nose, and throat may show such classic signs of allergy as "allergic shiners" or allergic creases at the edge of the nose.

While laboratory findings are certainly of importance in the establishment of a firm diagnosis of asthma, they assume particular importance in differential diagnosis and precise specification of the nature of the disorder in any individual case. Usual laboratory procedures include complete blood counts, nasal secretion and sputum analysis (in particular for eosinophilia indicative of allergy), chest x-ray (primarily to exclude other conditions), skin tests, direct challenges of the lung, exercise challenges, and pulmonary function tests.

Skin tests are often very useful in defining those substances to which a person might be lung sensitive. False negatives are very rare; that is, allergic sensitivity of the bronchial tree almost invariably is associated with skin reactivity. The reverse, however, is not the case: the skin and other organs may exhibit allergic reactivity to an antigen that produces no effect when delivered directly to the lung. In these instances, bronchial challenges of the lung are employed. Unlike skin tests, which may be carried out safely in an office setting, bronchial challenges involve significant medical risk and usually are done under more carefully controlled conditions because of the possibility of severe or delayed asthmatic reactions that may require vigorous treatment. Two kinds of challenges can be used. The first involves antigens (pollen, molds, house dust, and the like) prepared in an aerosol for inhalation. Such challenges can be indispensible when history and skin-test data are equivocal or when it is desirable to unequivocally determine the extent of bronchial reactivity to a suspected allergen, for example, as the basis for instituting immunotherapy or as a prelude to the clinical recommendation of an environmental change that cannot be made easily. The second involves similar direct inhaled challenges of the lung with histamine or methacholine. Both substances cause, in asthmatics, bronchoconstrictive responses that are from 100 to 1000 times greater than those exhibited by nonasthmatic individuals. These tests are very useful for firmly establishing the diagnosis of reversible airways obstruction, when reversibility is not clear on clinical grounds alone, and for the longitudinal assessment of airways reactivity. Methacholine challenge results, for all practical purposes, can be taken as definitive when the test is negative. That is, though there are several conditions under which the test may be positive, including asthma, a negative result precludes the diagnosis of asthma with a very high degree of certainty. Controlled exercise testing can aid treatment decisions substantially and serve as a guide to activity recommendations for patients. Further, it can serve to clarify the diagnosis of asthma, since reversible bronchospasm following exercise is an almost universal finding in asthma.

Assessment of pulmonary function is the *sine qua non* in the thorough evaluation of the asthmatic. In particular, pulmonary function tests can aid materially in differential diagnosis, precise specification of pathology, establishment of clinical severity, and the evaluation of provocation tests and treatment effectiveness. These tests include the measurement of lung volumes, pulmonary mechanics, ventilation, regional gas distribution, and arterial blood-gas tensions. While many severe, chronic asthmatics manifest residual abnormalities even when asymptomatic, results of tests are most revealing during periods of acute exacerbations or at differing severity levels of the chronic condition. Of the aforementioned measures, the most useful on an ordinary basis are the tests of ventilation based upon a forced vital capacity into a spirometer, a device which measures expired volume over time. The procedure involves having the patient exhale as much air as possible into the spirometer at maximum force following a full inhalation. From the outcome a number of measures can be obtained, the most important of which are the forced expiratory volume in one second (FEV, the volume expired in the first second), the peak expiratory flow rate (PEFR, the highest flow rate obtainable during forced expiration) and the maximum mid-expiratory flow rate (MMEF, the maximum flow rate obtained between 25 percent and 75 percent of the total expired volume). FEV and PEFR are highly dependent upon patient effort (i.e., whether the patient blows as hard as possible into the spirometer) and are primarily sensitive to large-airway obstruction. Because the site of obstruction in asthma may be in either the large or the small airways or both, measures that are differentially sensitive to the central (large) and peripheral (small) airways are necessary. The MMEF is both relatively effort independent and quite sensitive to small-airway pathology. An effort-independent, large-airway measurement is more complicated than such flow measures as airways resistance or its reciprocal, airways conductance. This measure can be derived in several ways but is most commonly obtained from a whole-body plethysmograph. The most useful lung volume measures, such as the functional residual capacity and residual volume, are obtained from this large and expensive instrument. These are primarily measures of small airways. While the aforementioned measurements provide excellent information, when the equipment is available, the most generally useful device is the portable PEFR meter (the Wright). Because of its favorable size, cost, and ease of use, it can be employed effectively in the office and also at home by the patient. Furthermore, the portable PEFR meter can yield very frequent measurement of lung function. In most cases, the PEFR will provide all of the pulmonary functional information that is ever necessary for most aspects of clinical diagnosis and treatment evaluation. However, as the sole measure for research purposes, the effort-dependent nature and exclusive sensitivity to large airways of the PEFR may present problems. In most research contexts, other measures, such as those described previously, must be employed. Nevertheless, there are few pulmonary functional measures other than the PEFR that are as practical to obtain on a daily basis.

Regional gas distribution determination can be made by the closing volume method, helium equilibration, or single-breath nitrogen washout techniques. These are used only in specialized circumstances and need not be described further here. The same is true of the many other measurements that can be obtained from the spirogram and the flow–volume curve. They too, however, become useful under less-than-ordinary conditions. Arterial oxygen and carbon dioxide tensions are not obtained routinely but often become crucial during the life-saving clinical evaluation and treatment of very severe asthma.

Treatment

Therapy for asthma almost always is directed toward one overriding goal: a therapeutic approach that provides as much control of symptoms as is possible with as little therapy (mainly medication) as is necessary, such that both the disease and its treatment interfere minimally with a productive and rewarding lifestyle. With few exceptions the drugs used to treat asthma possess varying degrees of disturbing, and in some cases dangerous, side-effects. As will become evident from the following discussion, the hope that behavioral intervention might reduce significantly, or in some cases even eliminate, the need for drugs in the treatment of asthma as yet has failed to materialize to any clinically significant extent. It also will become evident that, even though the behavioral specialists still have a vital role to play in the treatment of asthma, behavioral strategies rarely if ever will represent the primary therapeutic modality. Behavioralists invariably will find themselves working with secondary, albeit often highly important, problems associated with the disorder and its medical treatment. In the paragraphs that follow, the medical management of asthma will be characterized briefly, to be followed in subsequent sections by more in-depth discussion of the role of psychological variables in asthma and the behavioral strategies that can be employed along with appropriate medical management in the overall treatment of bronchial asthma.

Asthma may be manifested clinically by as little as a few mild attacks in a lifetime to severe, life-threatening, chronic asthma that responds only to the most vigorous therapy involving powerful drugs on a virtually continuous basis. Most asthmatics, however, fall somewhere in between, from seasonal asthma, requiring sustained therapy only at certain times during the year, to moderate perennial asthma, requiring year-round therapy. The rational therapeutic regimen must be tailored carefully to each case, in accord with diagnostic findings. The drugs available to the physician fall into three broad categories: bronchodilators, corticosteriods (whose mechanism of action is to date essentially unknown), and others (mainly cromolyn sodium, whose precise mechanism of action is also largely a matter of speculation). Also available are methods such as immunotherapy, the role of which will be described in turn.

Five classes of clinical manifestation are distinguished for therapeutic purposes: (1) mild sporadic episodes; (2) moderate chronic asthma; (3) severe chronic asthma; (4) acute serious attacks, or breakthroughs from the standpoint of chronic management; and (5) status asthmaticus. The last represents a life-threatening medical crisis and will not be considered here, as successful management is designed to avoid this situation. Essentially, no additional drugs are available for the treatment of status asthmaticus, but appropriate steps must be taken to stave off or, in the worse instances, to deal with consequences such as respiratory failure and cardiac arrest.

The mild-to-moderate asthmatic with infrequent episodes tends to respond well to symptomatic doses of oral or inhaled sympathomimetics. These include isopreterenol and metaproterenol (predominantly a beta receptor agonist), which are catecholamine-like substances that produce bronchodilation by relaxation of bronchial smooth muscle. Theophylline compounds, which are bronchodilating drugs in the same general class as caffeine (i.e., xanthine), can be given orally on a symptomatic basis. In the mild-to-moderate asthmatic, these drugs usually are well tolerated with few significant side-effects.

Moderate chronic asthma or extended seasonal exacerbations usually require continuous therapy. Typically this will involve a round-the-clock (every 6, 8, or 12 hours) daily therapy with oral theophylline and, if necessary, oral sympathomimetics. In this case, side-effects are of greater importance: nausea, vomiting, and central nervous system overstimulation with the former and disturbing tremor with the latter. The dosage of theophylline, the most useful drug in the management of chronic asthma, must be titrated carefully on an individual basis, as the range between therapeutic effectiveness and toxicity is quite narrow and drug metabolism varies widely from patient to patient.

Chronic severe asthma frequently requires regular treatment with corticosteroids, usually prednisone, in addition to the regimens just described. The major problem here is to avoid as much as possible the suppression of normal hypothalmic-pituitary-adrenal axis function; hence, prednisone therapy every other day (to allow adrenal function recovery on the off-medication day) is preferred if symptom control can be obtained. If not, daily steroid therapy must be employed.

Serious acute attacks, or breakthroughs from the standpoint of overall management, usually require parenteral therapy. Typically this involves, on order of priority, subcutaneous epinephrine, intravenous aminophylline (theophylline), and I.V. steroids. Additionally, extended exacerbations in nonsteroid-dependent cases may require short "bursts" of steroid therapy for one or two weeks until symptoms are brought under control. Less severe, acute attacks in chronic asthmatics may require only spot treatment with an inhaled sympathomimetic.

Examples of other management strategies include (1) pretreatment prior to expected precipitant exposure and (2) prophylactic therapy with cromolyn sodium. The latter can assume in some cases an important role in the management of chronic asthma. In certain individuals it can provide protection against exercise-induced asthma, clinical benefit in allergen-induced asthma, and steroid sparing effects. Because it is difficult to predict the therapeutic contribution of prophylactic therapy in any particular case, it usually is given a therapeutic trial because the benefits sometimes can be significant. Exercise-induced bronchospasm also very often can be managed successfully by pretreatment with inhaled sympathomimetics.

In some cases other methods, such as immunotherapy or the familiar "allergy shots" (whose true effectiveness in asthma is still controversial), can be of benefit to the asthmatic. Because of the time and costs involved, some asthma specialists require that bronchial (as opposed to simply skin) reactivity be demonstrated (by bronchial challenge tests) before a course of immunotherapy, usually lasting from 1 to 3 years, is considered worth undertaking. At the present time, however, many allergists begin immunotherapy on the basis of often-marginal skin-test and history data alone.

The use of environmental control strategies, such as elimination diets, change of geographical location, elimination of pets, and the like, are obvious in selected cases where a clear link between stimulus and response is demonstrated. It must be pointed out, however, that careless recommendations in this regard can do more harm than good. Examples include giving up a beloved pet, changing of many household articles, relocation with family or job upheaval, expensive and unusual diets, and expensive air-purification devices—without any convincing rationale or promise of success prior to the recommendation.

The final method that often is included in descriptions of therapeutic management strategies for the asthmatic—namely, behavioral techniques of various kinds—constitutes the general focus of the remainder of this chapter.

The Psychological Aspects of Asthma

Psychological Factors in Etiology

In general, the medical field conceives of asthma as basically an immunological disorder; however, the psychoanalytic formulations of French & Alexander (1941) dominates thought within psychosomatic medicine. These authors popularized the hypothesis that the origin of asthma was in the suppression of an intense emotion, specifically, "a suppressed cry for the mother." Until very recently the dominant theme among psychosomatic researchers has been that in some manner psychological variables play an etiologic role in asthma.

It may be instructive to provide a comparison between asthma and peptic ulcer. It generally is agreed that certain forms of psychological stress and conflict can lead more or less directly to increased gastric secretion in normal individuals. For persons who are on the high end of the gastric reactivity continuum, prolonged exposure to the appropriate forms of psychological stress ultimately may lead to ulceration of the stomach or duodenum. This analysis assigns a prominent role to psychological factors in the actual etiology of the lesion. While there surely exists a complex interaction between tissue susceptibility, normal gastric acid levels, secretory reactivity, and many environmental and psychological factors in the development of ulcer in any particular case, this formulation provides for the possibility that a lesion would not appear in the absence of sufficient psychological stress, even if all of the other factors were favorable to ulcer development. As such, peptic ulcer would seem to be an excellent example of a truly psychosomatic disease.

In contrast, for asthma there is simply no convincing evidence that the pathophysiological characteristics of asthma must result in any way from psychological influence (Creer, 1978). The current view is exactly the opposite; that is, psychological disturbances can result from the continued battle with asthma, or indeed any chronic illness, and that, in some affected individuals, psychological influences such as emotional stress may contribute to the frequency and severity of specific episodes of bronchospasm. Hence, many authors (Creer, 1978), are taking the position that asthma should not be considered a psychosomatic disorder. There is good reason to be very sympathetic toward this view, as the concept of psychosomatic usually includes notions regarding an etiologic role for psychological events. The sustained belief that psychological variables contribute in any way to the cause of asthma only will continue to divert attention away from the more fruitful study of the role psychological influences do play in the lives of affected individuals. Equally as pertinent, the traditional psychosomatic view only furthers the destructive notion, held by most laymen and too many professionals, that asthma is "all in the head." Such a belief is monstrously unfair and often psychologically damaging to asthma sufferers and their families. It also can lead to a very dangerous clinical approach to therapy for persons who sometimes are severely ill for no "fault" of their own.

Psychological Factors in Manifestation

Family. It appears that psychological factors in the family constellation do play a role in the manifestation of the disorder in some cases, though undoubtedly not in its etiology. For years clinicians have noticed that some childhood asthmatics obtained symptom reduction or remission when separated from their families for one reason or another. In the late 1950s, Peshkin even spoke of "parentectomy" as a treatment for asthma in some children (Peshkin, 1960). The effectiveness of separation was evident in the significant number of children whose symptoms remitted abruptly when they were sent to residential treatment centers such as the National Asthma Center in Denver. It remained likely, however, that the benefits of leaving home for a time were due to alterations of the physical rather than emotional environment. In a landmark study, Purcell and his colleagues (Purcell, Brady, Chai, Muser, Molk, Gordon, & Means, 1969) controlled for physical environment effects by removing the families of asthmatic children to a hotel for several weeks while the child remained home under the care of an adult child-care worker. They found that for children whose asthma displayed "emotional" overtones, this experimental separation from their families produced small but statistically significant changes in a number of asthma measures. While these results implicated general family stress in the manifestation of the disorder, more specific attempts to verify whether "rejecting" or "engulfing" mothers cause asthma have met with lack of success (McLean & Ching, 1973), and attempts to dichotomize asthmatics along an emotional–organic continuum have not proved fruitful (Mattsson, 1975). Hence, a safe conclusion would be that such emotional factors account for a modest amount of pulmonary variance in a minority of asthmatics.

Personality. The hope that a specific personality pattern is found to be associated with asthma has been pursued even more energetically and with less success. As Creer (1978) pointed out, asthma sufferers were claimed at one time or another to be overdependent, hypersensitive, overly aggressive, and overly passive. They were found to be more neurotic than normals and to describe themselves in a less favorable light. In general, when comparisons are made with those who suffer from other chronic illnesses, differences disappear (Neuhaus, 1958). It now generally is conceded that the frequently obtained personality differences between asthmatics and normals are a result of the disease itself and probably are only manifestations of the presence of chronic illness. There is no evidence to suggest that unique personality factors contribute to the development of the disorder. All of the investigations in this area were experimentally flawed and entailed the conceptual risk in the field of deemphasizing the importance of the biological processes that underlie asthma.

Emotional Stress. Psychophysiological investigations yielded slightly more encouraging results (Purcell & Weiss, 1970). A common clinical observation, often supported by patient report, was that attacks sometimes appeared during, or seemed to result from, emotional stress. Certainly emotional arousal, such as anxiety, frequently accompanies asthma episodes. Accordingly, a number of attempts were made to precipitate asthma by employing emotional stressors such as disturbing films (Weiss, Lyness, Molk, & Riley, 1976), recordings of the voice of a patient's mother (Hill, 1975), and discussions or hypnotic suggestions of stressful life situations (Clarke, 1970). Generally such stimuli proved capable at times of producing changes in respiratory patterns and slight decreases in pulmonary flow rates but did not produce frank asthma. The effects were very modest, though usually statistically significant and appeared only in some individuals. These results did present a paradox, however. Since the cornerstone of therapeutics in asthma has been the well-established bronchodilating effects of beta adrenergic substances, the question arises as to why such episodes, accompanied as they are by sympathetic arousal, should result in bronchospasm at all. A possible answer was proposed by Mathé & Knapp

(1971) as a consequence of experiments that suggested that some sort of an adrenergic defect may be involved. They found that some asthmatics appeared to produce less than normal amounts of epinephrine as indicated by decreased urinary epinephrine excretion as a result of emotional stress. These results have not been replicated, however.

The Vagus. Attempts to demonstrate that asthma might represent a "vagotonic" disorder, or one characterized by a relative parasympathetic dominance, have generally been unencouraging; nevertheless, recent work by Gold, Kessler, & Yu (1972) has forced renewed interest in the vagus. They have shown that significant bronchospasm can result from mechanical stimulation of vagally mediated epithelial irritant receptors. Such reflex bronchospasm is presently held to be a likely cause of mechanically induced bronchospasm in humans, which often results from coughing, some airborne irritants, cold air, and the like. It is a distinct possibility that many examples of so-called emotionally triggered asthma attacks may be due to this mechanism. Only very indirectly do gasping as a result of surprise, yelling during anger, and crying or laughing accompanying acute emotional states represent "emotional" asthma.

Imagination. The work on suggestion, relaxation, and placebo effects remains the most compelling line of research indicating that psychological variables may play a role in the control of airways tone. A number of reports in the literature (Luparello, Lyons, Bleecker, & McFadden, 1968) have indicated that inhaled aerosolized saline can result in bronchoconstriction when the subject is led to believe that the substance is one to which she or he is known to be sensitive; moreover, the resultant increase in airways resistance can be reversed by another inhalation of saline believed by the subject to be a standard bronchodilator. The only failures to replicate these effects have employed insensitive measurement methods, a situation confirmed by the Luparello et al. (1968), again underscoring that such effects are probably real but indeed modest. In a series of experiments in our own laboratory (Alexander, Miklich, & Hershkoff, 1972; Alexander, 1972; Alexander, Cropp, & Chai, 1979), we showed that psychological relaxation can result in very small but statistically significant decreases in airways resistance, as well as a retarding of the natural increase in resistance that occurs when maintenance oral bronchodilators are withheld. Again, these effects, though replicated by other investigators, are modest. Finally, Godfrey & Silverman (1973) noted that premedication with placebo can lead to a significant reduction in the degree of exercise-induced bronchospasm.

Conditioned Responses. Beginning almost a century ago, the possibility that learning or conditioning may influence bronchomotor tone also has been studied. MacKinzie (1886) anecdotally described a woman who was said to develop wheezing from the sight of a paper rose under glass.

Nevertheless, during the ensuing nine decades there have appeared no convincing laboratory demonstrations of "conditioned asthma," but several writers have discussed the likelihood of conditioned bronchospasm (Turnbull, 1962). It remains an intriguing possibility that the circumstances under which naturally occurring antigen-induced bronchospasm or sympathomimetically provided relief may represent a standard classical conditioning paradigm. For example, Pavlov's dogs were caused to have a conditioned connection between bell and salivation by means of a bell being sounded shortly before food powder was blown into their mouths. After many such pairings of the bell and food powder, the bell alone was capable of producing the reflexive salivation. Illustratively for the asthmatic, the bell might be the visual and olfactory sensations associated with a weed, while the pollen would be the food powder. The bronchospasm in this case would represent the "reflexive" allergic reaction to pollen, just as salivation is the reaction to food. After enough pairings between weed and pollen, simply seeing weeds should be capable of causing some conditioned bronchospasm. Similarly, the stimuli immediately preceding the inhalation of a pharmachological bronchodilator soon should elicit some conditioned relaxation of bronchial smooth muscle.

Although the foregoing analysis may seem theoretically compelling, closer scrutiny reveals problems. These kinds of classically conditioned responses have in general proved to be unstable and hard to develop. With the exception of conditioned responses that are highly adaptive for the organism, such as taste aversions to toxins or fear reactions, classically conditioned connections tend to dissipate or extinguish very rapidly if the conditioned stimulus is not continually paired with the stimulus producing the reflexive reaction (Kling & Riggs, 1971). For our example this means that for every occasion in which weed stimuli are not actually associated with the presence of pollen or a sufficient quantity of pollen (thus producing a "reflexive" bronchial reaction), we will have an extinction or deconditioning trial. Furthermore, the actual model for our example is technically called *long-delay* or *trace conditioning*, an even more unfavorable set of circumstances for the development and maintenance of classically conditioned responses. While suggestion and placebo effects certainly can be interpreted as due, at least in part, to historical conditioning trials, it is not surprising that both these effects and examples of "conditioned asthma" have been so elusive. Careful analysis suggests that conditioned bronchoconstriction or dilation would tend to develop only infrequently and almost never to any great degree in any particular case. As we have seen, natural conditioning trials, which must be numerous and occur under optimal circumstances for conditioned reactions to develop at all, in most instances would be defused continually by natural extinction trials.

Biofeedback. Recently, the possibility of biofeedback-assisted learning (or volitional control) in the lung has been investigated. This work required the use of elaborate and very expensive instrumentation to provide almost breath-by-breath analysis and feedback information of airways resistance. Furthermore, the validity of the technique employed, forced pressure oscillation, has been severely criticized. These difficulties notwithstanding and with recognition of the problems, Vachon & Rich (1976) and Feldman (1976) reported what appears to be reliable but very small learned drops in respiratory resistance in a few subjects. It is becoming increasingly clear in biofeedback research that generally very elaborate experimental control procedures are required before any obtained visceral changes can be ascribed confidently to learned voluntary control (Miller, 1978). As yet, such controls have not been employed in this work.

Conclusions. Although much enthusiastic and dedicated effort has been expended by investigators with a psychosomatic orientation, no really persuasive evidence has surfaced in support of the long-held notion that psychological variables play any role in the etiology of asthma. Nevertheless, it may be acknowledged that psychosocial variables may to some degree be capable of affecting pulmonary reactions in some individuals and, for a minority of patients, possibly the clinical course of asthma as well. Pessimistic as this assessment may be, a dispassionate appraisal indicates that psychosocial factors exert at best only a comparatively minor influence on pulmonary physiology and thus have very few practical clinical consequences for the majority of asthmatics under most circumstances. Neither asthmatics in general nor any specific subgroups of asthmatics demonstrate particular susceptibility to the pulmonary effects of psychological stimuli (Mattsson, 1975). To be sure, the lungs of asthmatics are hypersensitive (i.e., more reactive) when they encounter various levels of physical bronchoconstricting influences, but the respiratory tracts of other persons also will react, albeit less dramatically, to similar chemical or mechanical insult.

Lung hypersensitivity presents an interesting and instructive model. When subjected to a chemical insult, the pulmonary response of a person who will experience symptomatic bronchospasm (i.e., an asthmatic) is potentiated. In other words, asthmatics exhibit a pulmonary reaction many orders of magnitude greater than the response of an individual who will never experience symptoms (nonasthmatic). It follows that respiratory sensitivity probably lies on a continuum from normal to extremely marked reactivity. The practice of distinguishing between asthmatics and nonasthmatics possesses distinct clinical and psychological utility. Treating asthma as a disease entity, however, probably masks the fact that the asthma syndrome may well represent a pathological exaggeration of any one of a number of normal processes in the lung. The apparent discontinuity between asthmatics and nonasthmatics is likely due in large part to the fact that pulmonary function generally must decrease at least 20 percent from normal values before *any* loss of function is detectable by either the patient or a physician without special measuring instruments. Likewise, to the extent that any apparent variation is real, it is quite probable that the degree of pulmonary sensitivity to emotional stressors will be found to vary continuously rather than discretely among individuals, and that trans-situational variance in susceptibility will be evident for any given individual as well.

Considering the complex interaction among exogenous/environmental, psychosocial, abnormal/normal, and pathological/physiological variables, our comprehension of bronchial asthma must become much more highly sophisticated before we are capable of more than guesswork concerning which specific psychological stimulus will influence the clinical course of asthma in any individual case at any given time. The nature of this problem is at once evident when we consider that past research has failed as yet to generate any substantial evidence of either consistent similarities or differences among asthmatics vis-à-vis psychological variables.

Assessment in Applied Asthma Research

Insofar as asthma refers to the obstruction of proper gas exchange in the lung, it is impossible to overemphasize the necessity of carefully and adequately measuring lung function in the evaluation of intervention outcome. Particularly for controlled experimental purposes, reliance on patient self-report or wheezing assessment (by stethoscope) is not sufficient, and all manner of misleading and incorrect conclusions can be reached regarding the stimuli or treatment procedures relating to changes in asthma symptoms.

Outcome assessment data can be divided into four basic categories: (1) pulmonary function measurements; (2) medication requirements; (3) asthma attack characteristics; and (4) general care requirements. In the first category, pulmonary functional assessment, several important matters must be considered. Because of the constantly fluctuating nature of asthma, long-term measurement should be on a daily basis (usually morning and evening). Measuring devices include the use of such inexpensive and portable instruments as a hand-held peak flow meter, supplemented every one to four weeks by more complete functional assessment including measures sensitive to the two major sites of obstruction, namely, the large (central) and small (peripheral) airways. Effort-independent measures of each site should be collected (e.g., small-airways MMEF; large-airways resistance or its more desirable variants, such as specific airways conductance), in addition to the more usual effort-dependent measures of large-airways function (PEFR, FEV, and so on). It always must be remembered that asthma is characterized by an episodic rhythm, producing symptom remission during which pulmonary functions may be quite normal, either completely or in part.

The second most valuable outcome assessment tactic, especially for individuals requiring maintenance drugs used on a daily basis, is the measurement of medication requirements. Although drug requirement measures are to one degree or another dependent upon a complex interaction between difficult-to-specify patient and physician behaviors and judgments, as-needed medications constitute much "softer" data because their use is largely up to the discretion of the patient. Since the amount and kind of medication can influence lung function and its symptomatic manifestations substantially, the interpretation of drug data is always made in relation to other measures, such as daily pulmonary function scores and asthma attack counts. A decrease in medication requirements in most cases will represent a beneficial outcome only if lung function and asthma frequency have remained relatively unchanged. Similarly, noteworthy increases in lung function and/or decreases in symptom frequency may be indicative of success only when drugs have not increased. These reciprocal relationships between lung physiology, asthma symptomatology, and medications always must be understood and appreciated. Finally, it is best to require that the type of medication be held constant as much as possible throughout an investigational period because of the great difficulty in establishing action and potency equivalents among different kinds of drugs.

The measurable characteristics of asthma attacks include frequency, attack duration, and severity estimates. Measurements of these characteristics rely almost exclusively on patient report, using essentially subjective criteria of characteristics that are very difficult to define. At the National Asthma Center we have on one occasion or another used telemetered chest sounds, very-high-frequency clinical examinations or lung function assessments, and observer reports of audible wheezing, all with little success.

Lastly, general care requirements include such things as emergency-room visits, hospitalizations, physician's office visits, phone calls to physicians, and medical-cost and productive-time-lost estimates. These all are useful when the time windows over which assessments are being made are quite long (several months or years), because these are generally very-low-frequency events.

Behavioral Methods in Asthma Treatment

The background material provided thus far should have made it quite obvious that to deal therapeutically in an effective manner with the ravages of asthma often requires the talent of both medical and behavioral specialists. The purpose of this section is to delineate the sorts of behavioral techniques that were found useful by those involved in the treatment and rehabilitation of children who suffer from asthma. Behavioral intervention methods have been employed in the therapeutic management of asthma in two distinct ways: (1) to alter the abnormal pulmonary functioning more or less directly and (2) to alter maladaptive asthma-related behaviors. The kinds of problems that are found in each of these categories and the behavioral strategies that have been employed to deal with them will be discussed in turn.

The Alteration of Pulmonary Physiology

We have seen, on the one hand, that there was historically a strong belief that psychological variables directly influenced lung function to a significant degree, suggesting the possibility of more-or-less direct behavioral manipulation of asthmatic responding. It is now clear that this presumption was, quite simply, incorrect. On the other hand, despite this fact and because the drugs used to treat asthma can have dangerous side-effects, it was hoped that the need for medications might be reduced by the addition of effective behavioral manipulations of lung function to the treatment armamentarium. Thus, early behavioral studies in asthma treatment addressed—and rightly so, given our understanding at the time—the application of behavioral strategies to the alteration of pulmonary function.

The methods that were intended to alter lung function in asthma included relaxation training, biofeedback, systematic desensitization, and direct operant conditioning. Of these, relaxation and biofeedback have received by far the most attention.

Relaxation and Biofeedback. The initial experimental study of effects of relaxation in asthma was reported by Alexander et al., (1972). In this study, 20 children were offered six sessions of brief progressive relaxation training while another group of 16 children (matched with the first group on age, sex, and as closely as possible on the severity of asthma) received an equivalent number of sessions during which they simply sat quietly. Immediately before and after each session, pulmonary function was measured by a peak expiratory flow rate meter. The main interest in this study was to investigate the immediate effects of relaxation on pulmonary functioning; hence, no attempt was made to assess the potential long-term benefits of the regular practice of relaxation. Results indicated a statistically significant average increase of 21.63 liters per minute for the relaxation subjects, representing about an 11 percent improvement in pulmonary function, compared to a nonsignificant mean decrease of 6.14 liters per minute for the children in the resting condition.

These results were replicated by Alexander (1972) with a new group of children comparable to those participating in the first experiment but employing subjects as their own controls rather than a control-group design. A unique feature of this study was an attempt to discover if there were any ways of predicting which child would be most likely to respond beneficially to relaxation. In particular, the major question was whether relaxation could be considered to be a simple extension of resting or inactivity. If so, then the response to resting might predict deliberate relaxation. The results were very similar to the initial study. The average amount of PEFR change during relaxation was 23.5 liters per minute, while during resting there was a nonsignificant increase of 1.52 liters per minute. The difference between these two values was statistically signifi-cant; however, no significant relationship was found between the response to sitting quietly or resting and the response to relaxation, a result suggest-ing that purposeful relaxation could not be considered simply an extension of resting. Finally, no other predictor variables were found, although many possible candidates were investigated.

Alexander, Cropp, & Chai (1979) undertook yet a third experiment in order to address several crucial questions left unanswered by the two previous studies. These questions included (1) Does relaxation affect effort-independent measures of both large- and small-airways function as opposed to simple PEFR measurement? (2) Does relaxation affect airways function after the actual relaxation period ceases? (3) Does relaxation provide a clinically significant effect, that is, greater than 25 percent functional change as opposed to merely 11 percent referred to baseline? The subjects were 14 children, each of whom participated in 11 laboratory sessions divided into three distinct phases: resting, relaxation training, and unaided self-relaxation as learned in the relaxation training phase. Each session consisted of a pretest pulmonary-function assessment followed by four posttests of pulmonary function, extending the period of careful observation to approximately 1.5 hours post-relaxation. Each pulmonary function testing involved measurement in the whole-body plethysmo-graph, followed by a slow vital capacity effort and two forced vital capacity efforts.

During rest, a persistent tendency for pulmonary function to manifest a consistent, and in most cases monotonic, decline from the pretesting occasion was found. This was assured because testing was initiated six hours subsequent to the last administration of maintenance bronchodilator; hence, pulmonary function was declining due to the absence of medication. In contrast, the average relaxation response was a statistically significant shift toward maintenance of functions at the pretesting level. Nevertheless, the effect was very small and again failed to approach clinical significance.

Several other studies investigating relaxation effects in asthmatic children have appeared in the literature since this work began. Tal & Miklich (1976) reported small but statistically significant increases, over pretest rates, in one-second forced expiratory volume, following each of three sessions of very brief "quasi hypnotic tape recorded relaxation instruction" in 60 asthmatic youngsters. In addition to short-term effects, long-term effects of relaxation also have been studied. Both short- and long-term effects were studied by Erskine & Schonell (1979) in a 13-week study of ten moderate-to-severe adult asthmatics divided into two matched groups. One group received four sessions of similar training supplemented by mental (autogenic) relaxation suggestions. FEV and subjective symptom scores were measured both before and after each treatment session and once per week during the three pretreatment and six posttreatment weeks. No differences were found on any of the measures over time or between groups, either before and after treatment or before and after relaxation sessions. Davis, Saunders, Creer, & Chai (1973) also investigated both short- and long-term effects in 24 asthmatic children divided among three equal groups: (1) progressive relaxation training, (2) relaxation training plus forehead EMG biofeedback, and (3) self-control. They provided no information, however, regarding how biofeedback was combined with the muscular relaxation procedures. The study was divided into three phases: (1) baseline for eight days, (2) five treatment sessions, and (3) a posttreatment assessment period of eight days. Before and after each treatment session, and additionally three times per day throughout the duration of the study, peak expiratory flow rate measures were obtained. No overall differences among groups were found, either in terms of immediate changes over sessions or between baseline and postassessment phases.

A similar study was reported by Scherr, Crawford, Sergent, & Scherr (1975). During an eight-week treatment program, 22 children received half-hour sessions of relaxation training three times weekly between the second and seventh weeks of camp, while a control group of 22 children received no extra attention whatsoever. As with Davis et al. (1973), just described, training consisted of progressive relaxation supplemented by forehead EMG biofeedback. Again, no specification was provided regarding the procedure used in combining the two methods. Peak expiratory flow rates were obtained routinely on all children three times daily, but not before and after each session. Children receiving the experimental relaxation program manifested statistically greater improvement in terms of average PEFR from the first to the eighth week of the study, as well as greater reductions in the number of infirmary visits, number of asthma attacks, and steroid usage. Still, the authors very prudently suggested caution in interpreting these findings, since no attempt had been made to control for the special attention given the experimental subjects. Moreover, the medical staff independently rated members of the control group as having more severe asthma than the subjects in the experimental group.

Both of the studies just reviewed used a combination of muscular relaxation and EMG biofeedback. Kotses, Glaus, Crawford, Edwards, & Scherr (1976) attempted to investigate the distinct contribution of EMG biofeedback training. They divided 36 asthmatic children into three equal groups: contingent feedback, noncontingent feedback, and no treatment. For experimental purposes, each noncontingent subject was yoked throughout the duration of the study (nine sessions over three weeks) to a randomly selected contingent feedback subject, and children in both groups were told to try to lower the feedback tone. As in the previous study, measures of peak expiratory flow rates were obtained three times daily on all children but not immediately before and after each session. Results indicated that children in the contingent feedback group manifested a statistically significant increase in weekly mean PEFR compared to children in the noncontingent and no-treatment groups, who did not differ from each other. EMG data indicated decreased frontalis muscle tension for the feedback subjects, relative to increased muscle tension in the noncontingent group. There are two major difficulties with this study. First, as in the Scherr et al. (1975) experiment just described, the no-treatment group was not controlled for the extra attention given to experimental subjects. Although it may appear that the noncontingent yoked control group controlled for this variable as well as for the presence of the contingent feedback stimulus, more careful scrutiny reveals this probably was not the case at all. Because subjects in both groups were told to attempt to lower feedback tone (that is, to control forehead muscle activity), noncontingent subjects were presented in reality with an impossible task. While this instruction is fine for subjects receiving true contingent feedback, noncontingent subjects can discover easily that the feedback stimulus bears no relationship whatever to muscle tension or indeed to anything about their behavior, and thus they can realize that the task is hopeless relative to the instruction presented to them. As discussed by Alexander, White, & Wallace (1977), this can result in a countermotivated situation in which frustration and even anger are prominent features and where performance suffers accordingly. It is therefore hardly surprising that subjects in the noncontingent group manifested an increase in frontalis muscle tension during sessions and experienced no "relaxing" effect as measured by PEFR changes.

The Davis et al. (1973), Scherr et al. (1975), Kotses et al. (1976), and

Erskine & Schonell (1979) investigations all addressed a rather different question from that addressed by the three experiments by Alexander and his colleagues; namely, the effect of regular relaxation practice extending over periods of several weeks on frequent measures of pulmonary function obtained at times other than before and after the relaxation sessions. However, Davis and her colleagues (1973) and Erskin & Schonell (1979) studied both immediate and long-term effects of relaxation, finding no evidence for long-range effectiveness, whereas the other two studies found small but statistically significant increases in average peak expiratory flow rates over several weeks of training. While it is tempting to interpret the latter results as suggesting that the regular practice of relaxation may have long-range benefits, the lack of attention placebo control and the other methodological problems in these studies preclude the acceptance of this conclusion. When attention placebo control was included, Davis et al. (1973) found that long-term benefits failed to materialize and Erskin & Schonell (1979) simply found no effects of relaxation at all. It is impossible to conclude that either biofeedback alone or relaxation in conjunction with, or supplemented by, frontalis EMG biofeedback is an effective "relaxation" technique with which to bring about changes in pulmonary function for asthmatic children. Other research, albeit on nonasthmatic adults (Alexander, 1975; Alexander et al., 1977, Alexander & Smith, 1979), indicated rather clearly that EMG biofeedback procedures should not be considered an effective relaxation training method. Thus, overall, it now must be accepted that the evidence points securely toward the conclusion that no relaxation method of any kind has a clinically significant effect on pulmonary physiology in childhood or, for that matter, in adult asthmatics.

Of the two reports on airways resistance biofeedback that were mentioned (Vachon & Rich, 1976; Feldman, 1976) only the Feldman study employed children as subjects. Because of the elaborate and expensive equipment requirements and the marginal results obtained, biofeedback methods seem not to have received any further attention. This lack of enthusiasm is entirely justifiable in relation not only to the uninspiring results with asthmatics, but with regard to the rather discouraging state of affairs in biofeedback research generally, especially with autonomically mediated responses. The only other attempt to use a biofeedback treatment model with asthmatic individuals was reported by Tiep (1976), who cited clinical experience with simultaneous feedback given to the patient regarding the output of an electronic stethoscope as it monitored wheezing chest sounds. This method, however, has not generated any controlled laboratory research.

Systematic Desensitization. This was the first behavioral technique employed in the hope that a behavioral method could be found that would be capable of altering lung function. The rationale for the use of systematic desensitization treatment in asthma—which we now know is quite in error as far as asthma goes—was as follows: The "psychosomatic" asthma symptoms were considered to represent persistent, conditioned anxiety responses whose effects were manifested, at least in part, as an exaggerated reaction in a biologically vulnerable target organ, namely, the lung. It was reasoned that if the asthma was thus being mediated by anxiety, systematic desensitization should be therapeutically effective in reducing the conditioned anxiety and hence the wheezing. In the early sixties, when this formulation was proposed, there was considerable justification for it to be considered a highly sophisticated conceptualization as compared to the psychoanalytic notions of a child with a severe dependence conflict wheezing out for mother.

Several studies of increasingly high quality were carried out in the ensuing decade on the potential therapeutic effects of systematic desensitization for asthma. The first report on the clinical effectiveness of systematic desensitization with asthma was published by Walton (1960), who reported the case of a 30-year-old man suffering from asthmatic episodes that apparently were precipitated by anger and resentment, as well as by anxiety. The patient was administered systematic desensitization supplemented by assertiveness training. On the basis of self-ratings only, the patient's asthma reportedly improved commensurately with improvements in his social relationships.

The next report was provided by Cooper (1964), who treated a 24-year-old intrinsic asthmatic woman. Cooper initially hypothesized that the woman's asthma was psychosomatic in origin (i.e., represented a conditioned anxiety response), but, since specific anxiety-inducing stimuli could not be detected, Cooper hypothesized that stimulus generalization was responsible. A variant of systematic desensitization was used, consisting of deep-muscle relaxation (the anxiety inhibitor) in conjunction with deliberate evocation of anger and excitement by appropriate direct verbal suggestion. As with Walton's case (1960), the only measure of asthma was the patient's self-report, but Cooper reported that treatment was successful, noting that "training the patient to relax in traumatic situations has effectively raised her 'stress threshold' and rendered her relatively immune to asthmatic attacks precipitated by anxiety" (1964, p. 355).

Although the pioneering state of these two case studies must be acknowledged, their value is rather limited for several reasons. First, both reports failed to provide a firm medical diagnosis of asthma. Second, the outcome index consisted exclusively of patient self-reports in each case. Third, these reports also can be criticized on heuristic grounds: specifically, the rationale underlying therapy was that the asthmatic episodes were mediated by anxiety, an assumption that we are now quite certain is incorrect.

The first controlled clinical investigation of the efficacy of systematic desensitization in asthma treatment was reported by Moore (1965). She compared systematic desensitization, relaxation alone, and relaxation training supplemented by suggestions of symptom remission. Although differences among the three groups on subjective measures of symptomatology were not found, Moore did report a small yet statistically significant mean improvement in respiratory function in the group treated with systematic desensitization. This study is noteworthy in that it was the first report of any kind to include pulmonary-function assessment in addition to some measure of experimental control. While Moore is certainly to be commended, there is nevertheless a major problem, namely, measurement of respiratory function on a weekly basis only. Because of the highly intermittent nature of asthma, such a relatively infrequent measurement of peak expiratory flow rate does not permit any reliable conclusions to be drawn concerning either immediate clinical benefits or the long-term advantages of treatment (Chai, Purcell, Brady, & Falliers, 1968).

The most definitive test of the effectiveness of systematic desensitization was conducted with asthmatic children at the National Asthma Center in Denver. Miklich, Renne, Creer, Alexander, Chai, Davis, Hoffman, & Danker-Brown (1977) examined the effects of systematic desensitization, relative to a no-treatment control group, in a large-scale, long-term investigation in which the criterion index of clinical improvement was the one-second forced expiratory volume (FEV), measurements of which were collected twice daily throughout the investigation. The study consisted of five phases: (1) a baseline of 16 weeks, (2) ten weeks of treatment, (3) a nine-week posttreatment period, (4) an interim period of 11 weeks' duration during which no data were collected, and (5) a follow-up assessment phase of six weeks. Twenty-six severely asthmatic children were assigned to either systematic desensitization or no-treatment control. Pulmonary measurements were supplemented by data on frequency and type of medications taken, frequency of hospital admissions, and severity of daily symptoms. Results indicated an extremely small but statistically significant difference between groups on morning FEV only; however, this difference was attributable to attenuated rates of flow in control subjects rather than significant respiratory improvement in those patients receiving treatment. Thus, systematic desensitization failed to provide lasting therapeutic effects on pulmonary physiology.

Operant Conditioning. There have been three attempts to operantly condition increased flow rates by positive reinforcement. Khan, Staerk, & Bonk (1973) provided a group of ten asthmatic children with five sessions of so-called "linking training," during which a continuous series of forced vital capacity measures was undertaken and individual efforts were reinforced by praise and a red light whenever a particular "blow" on the spirometer was greater than the immediately preceding one. Following this phase, the children received ten similar training sessions after mild bronchospasm had been induced experimentally by a variety of means differing from child to child. No data were provided regarding the success these children had in successively increasing flow rates, but comparison of baseline data with measurements ten months after completion of the training sessions indicated that the children who were "trained" were significantly different from ten other asthmatic children who had received no treatment or attention of any kind. They differed on amount of medication required, the number of emergency-room visits, and the number of self-reported asthmatic attacks. The authors conceptualized their procedures as "conditioning," which is rather presumptuous given the fact that no real specification of conditioning procedures was delineated, no data were provided regarding whether or not conditioning even occurred, and none of the necessary controls for a learning experiment was in fact present. The results obtained were themselves uncontrolled in relation to nonspecific, attention placebo effects.

In a similar but more carefully designed and executed study, Danker, Miklich, Pratt, & Creer (1975) found neither immediate nor long-term increases in flow rates as a result of contingent reinforcement for successively higher-force expirations. They also failed to find any overall improvement in a variety of other indices of asthma.

More recently, Khan (1977) reported the results of another experiment methodologically similar to his previous effort. In this investigation, the experimental and control groups each were divided into predicted reactors and nonreactors on the basis of pulmonary response to placebo suggestion like those employed by Luparello et al. (1968). Once again, conditioning was claimed to have transpired but was not demonstrated, and, as before, there were inadequate controls for the confounding effects of attention, length of contact, expectation, and suggestion. No differences were found between predicted experimental reactors and nonreactors. Curiously, the author interprets the results as demonstrating success for his rather peculiar treatment package, even though the control reactor group manifested as much change on all measures as the group exposed to treatment. As in previous cases, no pulmonary function measures were employed in outcome assessment.

The Alteration of Asthma-Related Behaviors

While the methods just discussed were intended to impact pulmonary physiology in the asthmatic, the aim of the techniques in this second category is to alter behavioral excesses and deficits that are related to asthma in one way or another. When conceptualized correctly, there should be no expectation on the part of the practitioner that an intervention aimed at an asthma-related behavior will significantly alter lung function in the asthmatic in any direct manner. There is no question that indirect effects on the manifestation and course of the illness are possible, for example, when an intervention successfully increases compliance with a medical treatment procedure, which is directly aimed at symptom control (e.g., drug therapy). Nevertheless, it cannot be overemphasized that the behavioral clinician should, in all practical circumstances, avoid any temptation to believe or suggest to others that a behavioral intervention can be thought of as a primary treatment modality in asthma symptom (e.g., wheezing) control. This in no way relegates behavioral treatments in asthma to a permanently secondary status. Cases in which behavioral problems are clearly initial are not infrequent. These can occur when the pulmonary pathology is either potentially or in fact under good control but a behavioral difficulty is present that is precluding what would otherwise be uncomplicated medical management, for example, in cases of compliance problems and some cases of asthma-related fears.

Common behavioral excesses in asthma include, but certainly are not limited to, asthma panic, anxiety-induced hyperventilation, malingering, and inappropriate coughing.

Asthma Panic. Anxiety and fear responses that become associated (conditioned) to asthma-relevant stimuli have been called "asthma panic." These result as a direct consequence of extremely frightening, life-threatening episodes, where the fear may result from severe dyspnea and hypoxia; the anxious and fearful reactions of family members, physicians, nurses, and other medical personnel during acute attacks; and the pain associated with treatment (e.g., venous and arterial punctures), among other salient aspects of a medical crisis. While there is no evidence that the emotional state itself ever makes lung function worse directly, many indirect manifestations exist to the detriment of the asthmatic condition considered as a whole. For example, these fears can cause compliance problems and thus can exacerbate and/or prolong the attack. The result of this may lead to increased psychological and physical discomfort for the patient, both immediately and over extended periods of time.

There is currently a strong and well-deserved consensus that any of the deconditioning therapies (for example, systematic desensitization) represent the treatments of choice for clinical phobias (conditioned emotional reactions) in both children and adults. Hence, fear associated with asthma should be eminently treatable by these behavior therapies. In fact, this seems to be the case. At the National Asthma Center in Denver, numerous cases of asthma panic in youngsters have been treated successfully over the past ten years with systematic desensitization and its variants (*in vivo* desensitization and emotive imagery) and implosion (flooding). In no case was there the intention of altering lung function, and treatment success consisted strictly of reduced anxiety judged solely on clinical criteria such as subjective reports of improvement by the patient or observations by nurses, physicians, and others involved in the care of the individuals treated. Characteristic procedures are described in detail by Alexander (1977).

Hyperventilation. A widely appreciated clinical concommitant of anxiety is hyperventilation (Suess, Alexander, Smith, Sweeney, & Marion, 1980). This may be especially true in people with pulmonary problems who are thus sensitized to breathing difficulty. Both the hyperpnea (overly rapid breathing) and the hypocapnia (low arterial carbon dioxide tension) that characterize hyperventilation are bronchoconstrictors. Thus, anxiety-driven hyperventilation can be a serious problem in the asthmatic. In most cases treatment is twofold. First, it must be made clear to the patient that he or she is hyperventilating and that this respiratory pattern is inappropriate, can exacerbate bronchospasm, and can cause feelings of dyspnea beyond those attributable to the asthma alone. Second, relaxation responses to be used during the asthmatic episode are taught as an alternative behavior. Equivalently, systematic desensitization can be employed where there exists a link between the anxiety/hyperventilation response and asthma-relevant stimuli. The latter case, of course, simply represents an example of asthma panic that includes hyperventilation as a prominent response component.

Malingering. This presents a problem in asthma, especially with children, and there are well-documented behavioral treatment strategies to deal with it. This maladaptive behavior, which may develop in any chronically ill person, understandably may be shaped and maintained by a family or hospital staff who have seen a patient during a frightening, life-threatening attack. Because malingering often is reinforced by additional attention and care, a tactic that has been used successfully in its treatment is time-out from positive reinforcement. Creer and his colleagues (Creer, 1970; Creer, Weinberg, & Molk, 1974) have provided two reports of the use of time-out procedures to treat malingering in asthmatic children who were residential patients at the National Asthma Center. In each case, a reversal design consisting of baseline, time-out, return to baseline, and reinstatement of time-out contingencies was employed. During the treatment phases, each time the children requested inappropriate hospitalizations they were placed in rooms by themselves, with no TV, comic books, games, or other diversions. In general, the atmosphere was quiet, unstimulating, and appropriate for a "sick" child. Appropriateness of request for hospitalization based on medical need was judged by the admitting physician, who was blind to the presence of an experimental intervention. Also in each case, frequency and duration of hospital visits were dramatically decreased when the time-out procedures were in effect, compared to levels during baseline. No other indices of asthma were found to change during the period of investigation, underscoring the specificity of the treatment.

Using a procedure he called satiation, Creer (1978) reported a similar intervention in another case of malingering. First applied in a clinical setting by Ayllon (1963), the technique involved providing such large amounts of the reinforcer that it lost its reinforcing properties. In Ayllon's case, an institutionalized woman who hoarded towels was given more and more towels by hospital staff until she threw them out and stopped hoarding. Creer (1978) applied something like this strategy in the treatment of a young asthmatic boy. Behavioral analysis had revealed that this patient used demands for admission to the National Asthma Center acute-care unit as a mean of avoiding stressful events such as tests at school. After each brief hospitalization period of one day, the boy would claim he was well and request release. Treatment consisted of hospitalizing the child for three days rather than only one day each time he requested admission. During the eight months prior to the initiation of the procedure, 33 hospitalizations had occurred, in addition to 11 more during the month in which treatment was implemented. In the eight months following the procedure, there were only 12 hospital admissions. Evidence that the reduction in hospital admissions was a result of the procedures employed rather than a change in the severity or therapeutic control of the child's asthma was reflected by the total absence of changes in all other indices of asthma, such as medication requirements or daily lung-function tests. Whether or not one agrees that this procedure should be considered a reinforcer-satiation phenomenon, rather than a clear form of punishment, is less important than the fact that, like time-out, it works and works well.

Inappropriate Coughing. Cough is a common symptom in asthma. On occasion, however, it is manifested to a degree that is considerably out of proportion to that which is considered medically consistent with the severity of the illness. In these instances it can constitute an inappropriate behavioral excess that can become highly disruptive to normal individual and family functioning. Furthermore, coughing paroxysms, in themselves, can promote additional bronchospasm. Most often excessive coughing can be conceptualized as attention-getting behavior or simply as an inappropriate habitual pattern that is difficult for the individual to stop. Several cases of inappropriate cough in asthmatic children, treated by a variety of behavioral strategies, have been reported.

Neisworth & Moore (1972) reported the successful reduction of excessive coughing episodes in a seven-year-old asthmatic boy by employing a simple extinction procedure. The child's physician felt that the amount of coughing was inconsistent with the severity of his disease, and behavioral analysis revealed that parental attention probably was maintaining the coughing behavior, which occurred particularly at night. To initiate the intervention, the child's parents were instructed not to interact with their son once he was in bed. In accord with expectations, the procedure resulted in a systematic and rapid reduction in the inappropriate nighttime coughing behavior.

The removal of an aversive stimulus contingent upon the occurrence of the desired behavior is called *negative reinforcement*, while *punishment* is the application of an aversive consequence contingent upon the emission of an undesirable behavior. Aversive therapeutic methods usually represent the treatment of last resort, due to legal, humanitarian, and ethical considerations; however, in carefully selected cases, when used cautiously, an aversive technique can become the treatment of choice.

Alexander, Chai, Creer, Miklich, Renne, & Cardoso (1973) reported the treatment of a case of psychogenic cough, which combined both negative reinforcement and punishment procedures into the treatment. In this case a 15-year-old boy suffered from a chronic cough for 14 months prior to initiation of behavioral intervention. No organic basis for the cough could be demonstrated and extensive medical treatment attempts had failed. Behavioral analysis revealed a plausible conditioning history for the cough, and four specific cough precipitants were identified: the odors of beef grease, shampoo, hairspray, and bath soap. It was decided to treat the cough with a "response suppression shaping" procedure. In order to avoid a brief, 5-mA electric shock to the forearm, the patient was required to suppress coughing (the avoidance response) for increasingly longer periods following the controlled inhalation of a precipitating stimulus. The first precipitant required 75 conditioning trials. Fifty-one of these represented successful avoidance responses in that no cough was emitted within the critical avoidance interval. The remaining 24 trials included coughing that occurred during the critical interval, following which punishment was administered. Finally, the boy began to report no urge to cough following inhalations. The next precipitant required 60 trials to criterion, followed by 15 for the third precipitant, and finally, only one trial on the fourth. Only five days were necessary for the conditioning treatment. A prominent feature of this case was that the coughing had been maintained by contingent attention being paid to it by family members; however, simple extinction procedures, such as those employed by Neisworth & Moore (1972) described earlier, had proven unsuccessful. Indeed, much of the family's life had come to revolve about "the problem." The nature of the precipitating stimuli had required considerable accommodations in the eating and toilet habits of the family, a source of almost constant family disruption and stress. Finally, behavioral intervention at the family level was necessary to alter reinforcement patterns in order that coughing not be reestablished once it had been eliminated by the suppression procedure. There has been no recurrence of coughing in the more than nine years that have elapsed since the conclusion of treatment.

A punishment procedure also was employed by Creer, Chai, & Hoffman (1977) in the treatment of another case of chronic cough. In this instance, a 14-year-old boy was exhibiting almost continuous coughing for which, again, no organic basis could be determined. Here, too, extensive medical treatment efforts had failed. The coughing had become so persistent and disruptive that school officials found it necessary to suspend the boy from school until the problem could be resolved. Creer and his colleagues considered the coughing to be a learned response of unknown origin, but extinction procedures exhibited no effect. Because no specific precipitating stimuli could be isolated, a decision was made to employ a simple punishment method. Following baseline assessment, which revealed a very high coughing rate, it was explained to the boy that he was going to receive a moderate electric shock to his forearm each time he coughed. Dramatic results ensued. After only one shock, complete suppression of the response was attained. A three-year follow-up of this patient revealed neither recurrence of coughing nor the appearance of any other maladaptive respiratory pattern.

In the most recent application of conditioned suppression procedures, a 14-year-old asthmatic girl, who likewise exhibited a persistent chronic cough, was treated by Alexander (in press) at the National Asthma Center. As in the previous case, behavior analysis failed to isolate specific precipitating stimuli, and baseline observation revealed a rather uniform frequency of 10 to 15 coughs per minute during her waking hours. Prior to treatment the patient displayed volitional control over her coughing sufficient to reduce the baseline rate by approximately 50 percent. Conditioned response suppression, similar to that employed by Alexander et al. (1973) was used. Seven sessions encompassing 150 deconditioning trials were required to effect complete suppression of her maladaptive coughing. On only nine of the 150 trials did she fail to suppress coughing prior to termination of the systematically increasing critical suppression intervals, thus receiving a shock. A two-year follow-up has revealed absolutely no recurrence of her previous maladaptive coughing.

Behavioral and Educational Deficits.   Also common in those who suffer from asthma are behavioral and educational deficits of one sort or another. These can include (1) disruptions in normal intellectual and social development because of school and social disruptions, (2) the inability to comply with a medical regimen due to insufficient or incorrect information about asthma and its management, and (3) skill deficits in using therapeutic apparatus correctly. In some cases drug side-effects can result in interference with normal functioning.

Properly taking prescribed medications can present a major problem in treating any chronically ill patient. Many asthmatics use nebulized drugs that should be inhaled in a precise manner in order to be maximally effective for intermittent symptoms; therefore, the correct use of inhalants is an integral part of compliance to the medical regimen in asthma management. Renne & Creer (1976) addressed this problem by applying positive reinforcement procedures. They treated four asthmatic children who did not use correctly a device for administering a nebulized drug. This device automatically delivers a bronchodilating drug to the lungs under positive pressure. Employing a multiple baseline design across behaviors for experimental control, they taught all four children to use the machine by positively reinforcing successively closer approximations to proper utilization. Three responses (eye fixation, facial posturing, and diaphragmatic breathing) were trained sequentially. The success of this training procedure was documented by the reduced amount of drug required during subsequent treatments for relief of asthma symptoms. An advantage of this procedure is that it has been demonstrated to be successful when administered by hospital staff not trained in behavior modification. In a second phase of the experiment, nurses were taught how to employ the positive reinforcement procedure successfully with two additional children.

An educational deficit was treated successfully by Creer & Yoches (1971), using a response-cost procedure. Response cost is similar to time-out except that it involves the contingent withdrawal of a specified amount of reinforcement rather than the withdrawal of reinforcement over a specified time period. The amount of time spent attending to classroom materials was increased in two asthmatic children who had failed to develop these skills due to the amount of time lost from school because of illness. At the beginning of each classroom session the children were given 40 points, from which one point was subtracted (upon a signal from an observer) for each 30-second period spent not attending to classroom materials. Consistent with expectations, the children learned to retain the points (which could be exchanged for inexpensive gifts) and hence to increase appropriate attending behavior. As might be hoped, this generalized to the natural classroom environment and academic performance improved proportionately.

Recent research in the author's laboratory by a colleague, William Suess, has been aimed at delineating the extent to which the drugs commonly used to treat asthma may be contributing to deficits in intellectual functioning. At present, this research (as yet unreported) has focused primarily on possible learning and memory deficits caused by therapeutic corticosteroid medications. A second area of study is the concentration difficulties caused by the central-nervous-system-stimulating effects of the bronchodilators—such as beta adrenergic substances and theophylline—which are so indispensible in asthma management. Thus far, only the nature and extent of such deficits are receiving experimental attention, but the goal of this investigational program is the development of remedial strategies to counteract these iatrogenic effects.

Poor Coping Behaviors.   Finally, there is a complex of problems facing the chronically asthmatic child, just as there is for the victim of any chronic disorder, which can be characterized best as difficulties in adapting to and coping with a chronic problem. These difficulties were delineated in the description of the asthmatic child provided at the outset of this chapter. Problems such as poor self-concept, personal acceptance of the reality of having a chronic disease, development of an adaptive attitude toward the illness, adapting to the constraints and hardships associated with chronic asthma, and coping with the reactions of others to the presence of a chronic disorder all must be faced by the asthmatic. To a considerable extent the most effective therapeutic approach to this complex of problems appears to be education, primarily oriented toward the sufferer and her or his family. The asthmatic child in many respects ultimately must become an expert in the treatment of her or his own particular case. Probably the single most psychologically significant piece of information that can be offered to the asthmatic is that science now can confirm what the asthmatic has known for so long but in many instances has not been allowed to believe, namely, that asthma not only is not "all in the head" but is not even partly so. The behavioralist has a real stock in this effort, for the asthmatic only can be freed completely of this malevolent conception when the "head" experts also realize its lack of substance.

Conclusions

Asthma once was thought to be a definitive example of psychosomatic disease, namely, one in which psychological variables were thought to play a crucial role in both the etiology and symptomatic manifestations of the disorder. Four decades of increasingly careful and sophisticated research, however, have begun to change these beliefs substantially. Presently, the prevailing consensus is that psychological factors play no part whatsoever in the etiology of asthma and probably are relatively unimportant in the triggering of attacks in most, if not all, afflicted individuals. When emotional precipitation does occur, it is invariably due to asthma-producing physical behavior, for example, laughing, crying, or shouting, which can precipitate bronchospasms independent of the concomitant emotion. Nevertheless, precipitation of actual asthma episodes by psychological stress variables in the laboratory has remained an elusive goal. To date, some investigators have been able on occasion to produce small changes in lung dynamics as a result of the application of psychological stimuli, but, though these changes sometimes have been statistically reliable, they never have been coaxed into the range where they could be considered clinically significant. Psychological theories of asthma etiology, including conditioning theories, have fared very poorly. Most asthma specialists now feel that psychological difficulties can, and regularly do, result from having asthma but that there is virtually no persuasive evidence for an influence in the other direction. In most respects, the sorts of psychological development and adjustment problems caused by struggling with asthma are not substantially different from those that result from having any other chronic disorder.

A similar course has characterized the role of mental health specialists in the treatment of asthma. Psychological therapies have proven ineffective as a cure of asthma. Likewise, attempts to influence lung function directly and beneficially in asthmatics through psychological means have proven frustrating. Airways biofeedback, systematic desensitization, relaxation, operant conditioning, and other methods have not been able to produce therapeutically significant changes in pulmonary dynamics in those who suffer from asthma. It must be remembered that any positive claim of benefit to an asthmatic from any therapy, including a psychological one, must be substantiated by reliable pulmonary function measurement. Years of research have shown that assessment on any other basis (e.g., auscultation, clinical examination, patient subjective report, frequency of patient- and/or physician-defined asthma attacks, and medication usage when not defined by rigid criteria) can be and has been most deceiving in the hands of clinicians and researchers not specifically familiar and experienced with the disorder. In general, a review of the psychological literature in asthma reveals that the more recent the vintage of the experiment the less supportive the findings concerning direct effects in the lung for psychological variables and treatments. Most likely this represents an increase in rigor over time in both design and measurement in asthma experiments.

Given this assessment, is there a role for behavioral medicine specialists in the treatment of asthma? The answer is most definitely affirmative. Behavioral problems such as the adjustment to living with asthma, adjustment within families, compliance with treatment regimen, and anxieties and fears associated with asthma attacks themselves do, as expected, abound in asthmatic children. Hence, quite properly, behavioral specialists now find themselves dealing with the consequences of asthma, rather than its cause. For example, systematic desensitization has proven remarkably effective in treating asthma-related fears but not in altering lung function. Similarly, behavior modification techniques in all their variety have been employed with great success in the management of an impressive array of asthma-related maladaptive behaviors. There now is no doubt that the adequate treatment of asthma requires knowledgeable, sympathetic, and sophisticated medical therapy and, for many victims, behavioral treatment of commensurate quality and impact. Historically, psychosomatic practitioners and the mainstream of the medical profession seemed to share little common ground in asthma, either conceptually or practically. One of the most refreshing trends discernible in the new behavioral medicine approach to asthma is that the physician and the behavioralist are beginning to view asthma in an increasingly similar fashion. The main beneficiary of this rapprochement is the asthmatic child.

Thus, on the one hand, we now are in a position to state with considerable confidence that continued attempts to alter lung function to a clinically significant degree through psychological means will result in little success. On the other hand, the contribution of behavioral intervention to the overall treatment effort with asthmatics should continue to be developed with vigor. The research reviewed here, and all the clinical experience, points securely to the proposition that the fundamental rationale of behavioral intervention in asthma should be rehabilitation. For some time to come, however, the most crucial step for behavioralists probably will continue to be the shedding of the misconception that psychological factors contribute to the appearance of asthma symptoms in any sense. Once free of this burdensome notion, the behavioral clinician will discover happily that demonstratively effective technologies currently are available for the treatment of behavioral problems in asthma. In the many areas where developments are still necessary, there is no longer any need to be shackled by shopworn psychosomatic theories whose major contributions have been the light shed by their own demise. In retrospect, this may not have been an ignoble fate. Much has been learned, and more remains to be discovered.

References

Alexander, A. B. Systematic relaxation and flow rates in asthmatic children: Relationship to emotional precipitants and anxiety. *Journal of Psychosomatic Research*, 1972, *16*, 405–410.

Alexander, A. B. An experimental test of assumptions relating to the use of electromyographic biofeedback as a general relaxation training technique. *Psychophysiology,* 1975, *12,* 656–662.

Alexander, A. B. Behavioral methods in the clinical management of asthma. In W. D. Gentry & R. B. Williams (eds.), *Behavioral approaches to medical practice.* Cambridge, Mass.: Ballinger, 1977.

Alexander, A. B. Asthma. In S. N. Haynes & L. Gannon (eds.), *Psychosomatic disorders: A psychophysiological approach to etiology and treatment.* New York: Praeger, 1981.

Alexander, A. B., Chai, H., Creer, T. L., Miklich, D. R., Renne, C. M., & Cardoso, R. The elimination of psychronic cough by response suppression shaping. *Journal of Behavior Therapy and Experimental Psychiatry,* 1973, *4,* 75–80.

Alexander, A. B., Cropp, G. J. A., & Chai, H. The effects of relaxation training on pulmonary mechanics in children with asthma. *Journal of Applied Behavioral Analysis,* 1979, *12,* 27–35.

Alexander, A. B., Miklich, D. R., & Hershkoff, H. The immediate effects of systematic relaxation training on peak expiratory flow rates in asthmatic children. *Psychosomatic Medicine,* 1972, *34,* 388–394.

Alexander, A. B., & Smith, D. D. Clinical applications of EMG biofeedback. In R. J. Gatchel & K. P. Price (eds.), *Clinical applications of biofeedback; Appraisal and status.* New York: Pergamon Press, 1979.

Alexander, A. B., White, P. D., & Wallace, H. M. Training and transfer of training effects in EMG biofeedback assisted muscular relaxation. *Psychophysiology,* 1977, *14,* 551–559.

American Hospital Association. Figures on expense per patient day; section on hospital statistics, statistical tables. *Journal of the American Hospital Association,* 1971, *45,* 462.

Ayllon, T. Intensive treatment of psychotic behavior by stimulus satiation and food reinforcement. *Behavior Research and Therapy,* 1963, *1,* 53–61.

Chai, H., Purcell, K., Brady, L., & Falliers, C. J. Therapeutic and investigational evaluation of asthmatic children. *Journal of Allergy,* 1968, *41,* 23–36.

Clarke, P. S. Effects of emotion and cough on airways obstructions in asthma. *Medical Journal of Australia,* 1970, *1,* 535–539.

Cooper, A. J. A case of bronchial asthma treated by behavior therapy. *Behavior Research and Therapy,* 1964, *1,* 351–356.

Cooper, B. The economic costs of selected respiratory diseases, 1972. Unpublished report prepared for the Division of Lung Diseases Task Force on Prevention, Control and Education in Respiratory Diseases, 1976.

Creer, T. L. The use of time-out from positive reinforcement procedure with asthmatic children. *Journal of Psychosomatic Research,* 1970, *14,* 117–120.

Creer, T. L. Asthma: Psychological aspects and management. In E. Middleton, C. Reed, & E. Ellis (eds.), *Allergy: Principles and practice.* St. Louis: C. V. Mosby, 1978.

Creer, T. L., Chai, H., & Hoffman, A. A single application of an aversive stimulus to eliminate chronic cough: A case of one-trial learning. *Journal of Behavior Therapy and Experimental Psychiatry,* 1977, *8,* 107–109.

Creer, T. L., Weinberg, E., & Molk, L. Managing a hospital behavior problem:

Malingering. *Journal of Behavior Therapy and Experimental Psychiatry*, 1974, *5*, 259–262.

Creer, T. L. & Yoches, C. The modification of an inappropriate behavioral pattern in asthmatic children. *Journal of Chronic Diseases*, 1971, *24*, 507–513.

Danker, P. S., Miklich, D. R., Pratt, C., & Creer, T. L. An unsuccessful attempt to instrumentally condition peak expiratory flow rates in asthmatic children. *Journal of Psychosomatic Research*, 1975, *19*, 209–213.

Davis, D. J. NIAID Initiatives in allergy research. *Journal of Allergy and Clinical Immunology*, 1972, *49*, 323–328.

Davis, M. H., Saunders, D. R., Creer, T. L., & Chai, H. Relaxation training facilitated by biofeedback apparatus as a supplemental treatment in bronchial asthma. *Journal of Psychosomatic Research*, 1973, *17*, 211–218.

Edfors-Lubs, M. L. Allergy in 7000 twin pairs. *Acta Allergologica*, 1971, *26*, 249–285.

Erskine, J. & Schonell, M. Relaxation therapy in bronchial asthma. *Journal of Psychosomatic Research*, 1979, *23*, 131–139.

Feldman, G. M. The effect of biofeedback training on respiratory resistance of asthmatic children. *Psychosomatic Medicine*, 1976, *38*, 27–34.

French, T. M., & Alexander, F. Psychogenic factors in bronchial asthma. *Psychosomatic Medicine Monograph*, 1941, *4*, 2–94.

Godfrey, S., & Silverman, M. Demonstration of placebo response in asthma by means of exercise testing. *Journal of Psychosomatic Research*, 1973, *17*, 293–297.

Gold, W. M., Kessler, G. R., & Yu, D. Y. C. Role of vagus nerves in experimental asthma in allergic dogs. *Journal of Applied Physiology*, 1972, *33*, 719–725.

Hill, E. Bronchial reactions to selected psychological stimuli and concomitant autonomic activity and asthmatic children. Unpublished Ph.D. dissertation; Psychology Department, State University of New York at Buffalo, September 1975.

Khan, A. U. Effectiveness of biofeedback and counter-conditioning in the treatment of bronchial asthma. *Journal of Psychosomatic Research*, 1977, *21*, 97–104.

Khan, A. U., Staerk, M., & Bonk, C. Role of counter-conditioning in the treatment of asthma. *Journal of Psychosomatic Research*, 1973, *17*, 389–392.

Kling, J. W., & Riggs, L. A. (Eds.), Woodworth and Scholsberg's *Experimental Psychology* (3rd ed.) New York: Holt, Rinehart, and Winston, 1971.

Kotses, H., Glaus, K. D., Crawford, P. L., Edwards, J. E., & Scherr, M. S. Operant reduction of frontalis EMG activity in the treatment of asthma in children. *Journal of Psychosomatic Research*, 1976, *20*, 453–459.

Luparello, T., Lyons, H. A., Bleecker, E. R., & McFadden, E. R., Jr. Influences of suggestion on airway reactivity in asthmatic subjects. *Psychosomatic Medicine*, 1968, *30*, 819–825.

MacKinzie, J. N. The production of the so-called "rose-cold" by means of an artificial rose, with remarks and historical notes. *American Journal of Medical Science*, 1886, *91*, 45–57.

Mathé, A. A., & Knapp, P. H. Emotional and adrenal reactions to stress in bronchial asthma. *Psychosomatic Medicine*, 1971, *33*, 323–338.

Mattsson, A. Psychologic aspects of childhood asthma. *Pediatric Clinics of North America*, 1975, *22*, 77–88.

McLean, J. A., & Ching, A. Y. T. Follow-up study of relationships between family situation and bronchial asthma in children. *Journal of the American Academy of Child Psychiatry*, 1973, *12*, 142–161.

Miklich, D. R., Renne, C. M., Creer, T. L., Alexander, A. B., Chai, H., Davis, M. H., Hoffman, A., & Danker-Brown, P. The clinical utility of behavior therapy as an adjunctive treatment for asthma. *Journal of Allergy and Clinical Immunology*, 1977, *60*, 285–294.

Miller, N. E. Biofeedback and visceral learning. In M. R. Rosenzweig & L. W. Porter (eds.), *Annual Review of Psychology*. Palo Alto, Calif.: Annual Reviews, 1978.

Moore, N. Behavior therapy in bronchial asthma: A controlled study. *Journal of Psychosomatic Research*, 1965, *9*, 257–276.

National Center for Health Statistics. Chronic conditions and limitations of activity and mobility in the United States, July 1965–July 1967. *Vital and Health Statistics*, 1971, Series 10, No. 61.

Neisworth, J. T. & Moore, F. Operant treatment of asthmatic responding with the parent as therapist. *Behavior Therapy*, 1972, *3*, 95–99.

Neuhaus, E. C. A personality study of asthmatic and cardiac children. *Psychosomatic Medicine*, 1958, *20*, 181–186.

Peshkin, M. M. Management of the institutionalized child with intractable asthma. *Annals of Allergy*, 1960, *18*, 75–79.

Purcell, K., Brady, K., Chai, H., Muser, J., Molk, L., Gordon, N., & Means, J. The effect on asthma in children of experimental separation from family. *Psychosomatic Medicine*, 1969, *31*, 144–164.

Purcell, K., & Weiss, J. H. Asthma. In C. G. Costello (ed.), *Symptoms of psychopathology: A handbook*. New York: John Wiley, 1970.

Rackeman, F. M. Studies in asthma: Analysis of 213 cases in which patients were relieved for more than 2 years. *Archives of Internal Medicine*, 1928, *41*, 346–369.

Renne, C. M., & Creer, T. L. The effects of training on the use of inhalation therapy equipment by children with asthma. *Journal of Applied Behavior Analysis*, 1976, *9*, 1–11.

Scherr, M. S., Crawford, P. L., Sergent, C. B., & Scherr, C. A. Effect of biofeedback techniques on chronic asthma in a summer camp environment. *Annals of Allergy*, 1975, *35*, 289–295.

Schiffer, C. G., & Hunt, E. P. *Illness among children: Data from U.S. national health survey*. Washington, D.C.: U.S. Government Printing Office, 1963 *(Children's Bureau Publication No. 405)*.

Segal, M. S. Death in bronchial asthma. In E. B. Weiss & M. S. Segal (eds.), *Bronchial asthma: Mechanisms and therapeutics*. Boston: Little, Brown, 1976.

Suess, W. M., Alexander, A. B., Smith, D. D., Sweeney, H. W., & Marion, R. J. The effects of psychological stress on respiration: A preliminary study of anxiety and hyperventilation. *Psychophysiology*, 1980, *17*, 535–540.

Szentivanyi, A. The beta adrenergic theory of the atopic abnormality in bronchial asthma. *Journal of Allergy*, 1968, *42*, 203–244.

Tal, A., & Miklich, D. R. Emotionally induced decreases in pulmonary flow rates in asthmatic children. *Psychosomatic Medicine*, 1976, *38*:3, 190–200.

Tiep, B. Biofeedback approaches specific to the treatment of patients with bronchial asthma. Paper presented at the Third Annual UCLA Seminar on New Approaches with Biofeedback, Yosemite, California, 1976.

Turnbull, J. W. Asthma conceived as a learned response. *Journal of Psychosomatic Research*, 1962, *6*, 59–70.

Vachon, L., & Rich, E. S. Visceral learning in asthma. *Psychosomatic Medicine*, 1976, *38*, 122–130.

Walton, D. The application of learning theory to the treatment of a case of bronchial asthma. In H. J. Eysenck (ed.), *Behavior therapy and the neuroses*. New York: MacMillan, 1960.

Weiss, J. H., Lyness, J., Molk, L., & Riley, J. Induced respiratory change in asthmatic children. *Journal of Psychosomatic Research*, 1976, *20*, 115–123.

CHAPTER 4

Elevated Blood Pressure and Blood Pressure Reactivity in Children and Adolescents

Thomas J. Coates, Ph.D.

Introduction

A chapter on elevated blood pressure may seem out of place in a volume on pediatric behavioral medicine. The question comes immediately to mind: Is hypertension a problem among children and adolescents? The answer is a matter of perspective. If blood pressure is not taken seriously until it exceeds some arbitrary criterion, such as 140/90 mmHg, then hypertension in children is relatively rare and usually secondary to some underlying pathology. When elevated blood pressure is viewed as a quantitative and not a qualitative disorder, when blood pressure is evaluated in relation to age-related and not absolute norms, and when tracking (the tendency of elevated blood pressure to persist) is documented carefully, then pediatric elevated blood pressure takes on serious dimensions. Young persons are not likely to experience the negative effects of elevated blood pressure as children or adolescents, but they are certainly at risk for developing essential hypertension as adults. The potential exists to modify the course of their elevated blood pressure and thus mount important primary prevention programs.

We will concern ourselves in this chapter with two phenomena: *basal blood pressure,* or that level of blood pressure obtained by averaging

Preparation of this manuscript was supported in part by grants #1-R23-HL 24297 from the National Heart, Lung, and Blood Institute and #1-R03-MH 35148 from the National Institute of Mental Health.

several separate measures, an average that is likely to be reproducible; and *blood pressure reactivity*, or acute rises and falls in blood pressure occurring in response to environmental stressors. Correlates and methods for modifying both will be presented in turn.

Diseases of the cardiovascular system are the leading cause of death and premature death in Western industrialized societies (Surgeon General of the United States, 1979; American Heart Association, 1976; Pooling Project Research Group, 1978). These diseases produce immense economic, social, and psychological suffering, even when they do not cause death. Prevention of cardiovascular disease is a key objective of health promotion. In *Healthy People, The Surgeon General's Report on Health Prevention* (Surgeon General, 1979), chronic diseases such as heart disease and cancer were singled out as priority targets. In relation to adolescents and young adults, it was stressed that ". . . although chronic diseases are not among the major causes of death at this period in life, the lifestyle and behavior patterns which are shaped during these years may determine later susceptibility to chronic diseases."

Adding to our understanding of processes related to increased basal blood pressure and to exaggerated blood pressure reactivity in adolescents is one arena of research that ultimately could prove beneficial in preventing cardiovascular disease. It might be possible to decrease the damage to the cardiovascular system that comes from persistent or acute increases in blood pressure if these processes can be elucidated. Cardiovascular diseases, including hypertension, stem from multiple etiologies. Behavioral, environmental, and physiological variables influence, at least in part, basal blood pressure and blood pressure response to stress. Further examination of these variables is important because they are potentially modifiable and changing them would influence blood pressure levels and responses to stress.

Arterial blood pressure is among the most important factors in increased risk for morbidity and mortality due to cardiovascular disease (Stamler, Stamler, Riadlinger, Algera, & Roberts, 1976). Hypertension left untreated inflicts damage on arterial walls, promotes kidney damage, and places a strain on the heart, which is forced to work harder in order to move the blood against higher-than-optimal pressures.

Blood pressure reactivity in young persons also may be a significant risk factor for the development of hypertension. It is postulated that hypertension develops in suceptible young persons who respond to environmental or emotional stress by high cardiac output, increased peripheral resistance, or both. When faced with a challenging stimulus, the organism responds with increased output of epinephrine and norepinephrine. The catecholamines cause a rise in peripheral resistance and cardiac output, and acute blood pressure increases result. Fixed hypertension may occur over time as acute increases in blood pressure cause progressive changes in anatomical structures and changes in blood pressure regulation mechanisms.

Measuring Blood Pressure in Children and Adolescents

Blood pressure is a state and not a trait. As with many physiological measures, blood pressure is quite labile, being responsive to a variety of environmental, cognitive, and physiological variables. Moreover, it is well documented that a variety of factors can influence the accuracy of any single blood pressure measurement. Beyond measurement error is the issue that blood pressure is variable with time. Multiple blood pressures are needed to average out variability over time. Insel & Chadwick (in press) reported that intrapersonal variability accounts for 20 to 30 percent of variance of blood pressure measures in adults, but 50 to 60 percent of blood pressure variance in children.

The issue becomes important when norms for evaluating blood pressure are examined. The Task Force on Blood Pressure Control (1977) published a monograph describing current knowledge, state of the art for treatment, and percentile grids for evaluating pediatric blood pressures. The norms (Figures 4.1 and 4.2) are based on data from three epidemiologic studies: (1) Muscatine, (2) University of Iowa, and (3) Rochester, Minnesota (Mayo Clinic). The data are based on single casual blood pressures taken shortly after the children were seated and the cuff was placed on their arms.

By contrast, data from the Bogalusa Heart Study (Berenson, 1980) are based on the average of 6 blood pressures taken in a relaxed manner over 20 to 40 minutes. Figures 4.1 and 4.2 present percentile grids from the Bogalusa Study overlaid on the norms from the Pediatric Task Force. The effects of repeated measurement in a relaxed atmosphere are obvious, as the Bogalusa norms are considerably lower than the Pediatric Task Force Norms.

Tracking

Casual measures and repeated measures both present different information about blood pressure. Neither index, in the abstract, can be regarded necessarily as more true or real than the other; however, because pediatric blood pressure is so variable, sampling theory would indicate that multiple measures are needed in order to eliminate variation due to occasion and in order to obtain a suitable index of variation in measurement (Coates & Thoresen, 1978).

Reproducibility of measures provides a second index for making choices

Figure 4.1   The 50th Percentile of Systolic Blood Pressures. Derived from the Task Force on Blood Pressure Control (1977) and from the Bogalusa Heart Study (Berenson, 1980). The 95th percentile for the older age group also is indicated.

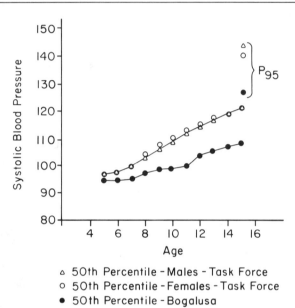

△ 50th Percentile – Males – Task Force
○ 50th Percentile – Females – Task Force
● 50th Percentile – Bogalusa

among measurement strategies. *Tracking* refers to the phenomenon that a person's relative status on a physiological index is relatively invariant; once elevated, blood pressure will tend to remain elevated relative to others in the population.

Level of elevated blood pressure during adolescence and young adulthood is predictive of later hypertension (Miall & Lovell, 1967; Paffenbarger, Thorne, & Wing, 1968; Harlan, Oberman, Mitchel, & Graybiel, 1973). In defense of using repeated measures, Harlan, Osborne, & Graybiel (1964), in their 13-year follow-up of 350 naval flight students, found that basal blood pressures predicted subsequent pressures in the same individuals better than did casual pressures: " . . . minimizing extraneous influences probably increases the validity and predictive capability of blood pressures recorded early in life."

Remarkable tracking of blood pressures has been observed in the Bogalusa study. Data from 3524 children aged 5, 8, 11, and 14 at initial examination were recollected one year later. The correlation between

Figure 4.2   The 50th Percentile of Diastolic Blood Pressures. Derived from the Task Force on Blood Pressure Control (1977) and from the Bogalusa Heart Study (Berenson et al., 1979). The 95th percentile for the older age group also is indicated.

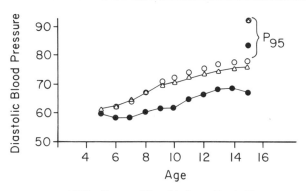

examination and reexamination was 0.70/0.50 (systolic/diastolic). Observations from a group of 35 fifth graders examined monthly were pooled to examine intrachild blood pressure and to estimate regression toward the mean. In a multiple-regression analysis, the previous year's blood pressure and an index of present body size accounted for 39 to 55 percent of systolic blood pressure variability, whereas the previous year's systolic blood pressure contributed a partial correlation coefficient of 0.60 to 0.70 for each age cohort. These tracking correlations are considerably larger than the .30 correlations obtained in the Muscatine study (Lauer, Filer, Reiter, & Clarke, 1976) and attest one more time to the need for repeated measures. These tracking correlations did not diminish in size as cohorts were followed across subsequent years.

Measurement Methods

Berenson (1980) suggests, for blood pressure measurement of children, strict guidelines designed to reduce error from several sources:

1. *Instruments.* Maintain at regular intervals; check and adjust mercury periodically; recalibrate periodically; use correct cuff sizes; apply correctly; use sensitive (bell or electronic) stethoscope.

2. *Examiner*. Check for hearing acuity; maintain eye level at mercury meniscus; keep patient's brachial artery at heart level; avoid venous engorgement.
3. *Examinee*. Void before examination; keep calm; space examinations every one to two minutes; get child to see other children being examined; take several measures.

Correlates of Elevated Blood Pressure among Young Persons

Identifying factors associated with elevated blood pressure might (1) enable us to identify populations at greater risk for elevated blood pressure and (2) help us to identify possible intervention targets. A comprehensive listing of variables that influence blood pressure follows.

Family History	Mother's blood pressure
	Father's blood pressure
	Siblings' blood pressure
	Mother's relative weight
	Father's relative weight
	Siblings' relative weights
	History of cardiovascular disease
Status	Sex
	Race
	Socioeconomic class
Ponderosity	Relative weight
	Relative fat
Maturity	Skeletal maturity
	Sexual maturity
Diet	Salt intake
Hemodynamics	Cardiac output
	Peripheral resistance
	Left ventricle muscle mass
Behavioral Factors	Type A (coronary prone) behavior
	Blood pressure response
	Cardiac output response
	Peripheral resistance response
Renal Function	
Hormone Function	
Mood	

Our discussion will be limited to those useful in identifying high-risk populations or possible points of intervention.

Family History

Family history of hypertension is one of the major predictors of hypertension. Paffenbarger et al. (1968), in their longitudinal study of precursors of hypertension in college students, reported that history of parental blood pressure contributed to the equation for predicting hypertension in later life. Zinner, Levy, & Kass (1971) extended these observations to a population ranging in age from two to 14 years, with a mean of 8.3 years. The sample included 721 children from 190 natural families. Maternal–child correlation coefficients were .16 for systolic and .17 for diastolic pressures; sib–sib systolic/diastolic correlations were .34 and .32, respectively. Within-family variance of children's blood pressure was significantly lower than between-family variance for both systolic ($F = 3.08$) and diastolic ($F = 2.68$) pressures, respectively.

Larger epidemiological studies generally have confirmed within-family concordance. Holland & Beresford (1975), for example, studied 501 families selected at random but stratified by family size and social class. The major determinants of blood presures in children five to eight years of age were parental weight and blood pressure. Children's blood pressures also were correlated highly with those of their siblings. Kass, Zinner, Margolius, Yhu, Rosner, & Donner (1975) extended the findings downward to a sample ranging from two to 14 years of age. They also studied the sample four years later and found familial aggregations that again were significant. Klein, Hennikens, Jesse, Gourley, & Blumenthal (1975) reported parallel results with black and white families. Langford & Watson (1973) reported similar correlations for diastolic blood pressure among full siblings aged 14 to 20 (.379) and among half-siblings (.354).

Feinleib, Garrison, Borhani, Rosenman, & Christian (1975) estimated that as much as 60 percent of the variance in blood pressure may be due to genetic factors. These estimates were drawn by studying 248 monozygous twins and 264 dizygous twins from five study centers across the country. Correlations among monozygous twins' blood pressures (.55/.58) are higher than the correlations found among dizygous twins (.25/.27). Using data from other studies to show the generally lower correlation among siblings, these investigators estimated relative genetic and environmental contributions to blood pressure using a simple additive model.

Genetic differences alone accounting for blood pressure variance may be questioned on two grounds. First, as Feinleib et al. (1975) pointed out, their results are derived from studying persons in a relatively homogeneous environment. Genetic variance might be inflated because environmental variance has been suppressed. Second, there is a striking similarity in sib–sib and parent–sib relationships found in many different ethnic groups and with different levels of blood pressure and potentially different physical and social environments (cf. Beaglehole, Salmond, &

Prior, 1975). Cassel (cf. Paul, 1975, p. 419) suggested that this finding supports the hypothesis that the distribution of genes responsible for blood pressure must be the same across societies and, therefore, cross-cultural differences cannot be explained by genetic factors alone.

In summary, there is little question that genetic factors are operative in elevated blood pressure and that controversies about the exact contribution of genetic factors will continue. The question does need to be reframed, however, so that the more important question is not obscured, namely, What interactions of environmental and genetic factors produce high blood pressure? The complexity of the phenomenon must not be obscured by the myopia of investigators with favorite but perhaps too-narrow hypotheses.

Status

Sex. Differences between the sexes in average blood pressures presumably emerge in late adolescence. Average blood pressures among adult males are typically higher than among adult females; this relationship generally holds true across racial groups as well (Stamler et al., 1976). The trends are less clear cut among young persons. The Task Force on Blood Pressure Control (1977) reported no blood pressure differences between males and females from two to 14 years of age. After the age of 14, however, average blood pressures and the prevalence of hypertension among males increased above the levels reported for females. Voors, Foster, Frericks, Webber, & Berenson (1976) also found quite similar pressures among males and females aged one to 15 years. Other studies with older adolescents have reported characteristic sex differences both among blacks (Dube, Kapoor, Ratner, & Tunick, 1975; Kilcoyne, Richter, & Alsup, 1974) and whites (Kotchen, Dotchen, Schwertman, & Kuller, 1974; Miller & Shekelle, 1976).

Race. Blacks have an unusually high prevalence of essential hypertension and related disorders in the United States (Finnerty, Shaw, & Himmelsback, 1973; Chenoweth, 1973). Average blood pressure readings for black males and black females exceed those found in white males and females; the prevalence of hypertension in black males is two times greater than that in white males and is associated with higher morbidity and mortality (Stamler et al., 1976).

Voors et al. (1976), in the Bogalusa Study, using six blood-pressure observations, found that black children had significantly higher blood pressure than white children. This difference became obvious beginning at age ten. The National Center for Health Statistics (1973, 1977) also reported small but consistent differences in mean diastolic pressures between black and white children aged five to 11 years. With sensitive measurements in large samples, characteristic racial differences might be detected among preadolescent children as well. Comstock (1957) found significant elevations among blacks aged 15 to 24. Kotchen et al. (1974) found significant racial differences among 18-to-19 year olds.

Other studies using casual measures found no differences. The Task Force on Blood Pressure Control (1977) reported no racial differences among two-to-five year olds. Differences may not emerge in middle to late adolescence. Kilcoyne et al. (1974), Miller & Shekelle (1976), and Schwartz & Leitch (1975) did not find differences between 14-to-19 year olds.

The distribution of pressures among blacks is displaced to the upper end of values in comparison to whites; more blacks than whites may show sustained elevations in blood pressure when rescreened a second time (Kilcoyne et al., 1974; Miller & Shekelle, 1976). Voors et al. (1976) reported that a significantly greater percentage of black children than would be expected by chance have blood pressures above the 95th percentile.

Socioeconomic Class. Lower socioeconomic class is associated with elevated blood pressure. Langford, Watson, & Douglas (1968), in a study of 5000 black students and 5500 white students reported higher blood pressures in rural than in city students and an inverse relationship between socioeconomic status and blood pressure among urban students. The usual black–white blood pressure differences were abolished when urban black upper-income girls were compared with rural whites, and this relationship also was reversed significantly in males when the same comparison was made. Kotchen et al. (1974) replicated these results among black students only. Inner-city blacks had higher blood pressures than blacks attending a racially integrated school in a middle-class residential area. Among blacks, higher blood pressures were found in children whose parents worked as laborers or were unemployed than in children of parents in professional occupations. Holland & Beresford (1975) reported inverse relationships among blood pressure and socioeconomic class in studying 501 London families.

Ponderosity: Weight and Overweight

Weight and weight status are correlated consistently with blood pressure across the complete distribution of blood pressures. Londe, Bourgoigne, Robson, & Goldring (1971) reported that the prevalence of obesity was higher in hypertensive persons (53%) than in normotensive controls (14%). Heyden, Bartel, Hanes, & McDonough (1969) found that an increase in weight was the only decisive factor in determining who was susceptible for the development of sustained hypertension. Those developing sustained hypertension at the seven-year follow-up had gained weight, while those becoming normotensive had not. Lauer and Bartner (1977) reexamined the

13 percent of those persons with pressures above 140/90 mmHg. One percent of the total sample retested above this level. Of this group, 50 percent were extremely obese. Among the six hypertensives who were lean, 50 percent were found to have hypertension secondary to kidney disorders or use of birth-control pills.

Blood pressures are higher among samples of obese persons than among samples of normal-weight persons. De Castro, Biesbroeck, Erickson, Farrel, Leong, Murphy, and Green (1976) studied 320 male high-school students. Using 20 pounds above mean weight for height as a criterion for obesity, the obese had average blood pressures of 124/80 mmHg, versus 116/73 mmHg for the nonobese. Court, Hill, Dunlop, & Boulton (1974) studied 109 obese persons 1.1 to 17.8 years of age who ranged from 3 to 113 percent overweight. The correlation between measures of subscapular skinfold and pressures were robust (systolic: males = .88, females = .78; diastolic: males = .80, females = .70). Coates, Jeffery, Slinkard, Killen, & Danaher (in press) reported significant relationships in 36 overweight adolescents (13 to 17 years of age; 15 to 100 percent overweight for sex, age, and height) among the factors of weight, percent overweight, and systolic blood pressure. The same relationships were found before and after the students participated in a program designed to reduce their obesity. Epidemiological studies have reported consistently that increases in blood pressure are correlated with increases in weight. These relationships hold true in black and white children and across the entire range of blood pressures and age groups (Lauer et al., 1976; Miller & Shekelle, 1976; Voors et al., 1976; Holland & Beresford, 1975; Dube et al., 1975; Stine, Hepner, & Greenstreet, 1975). Voors et al. (1976) found that the ponderosity index consistently entered first in stepwise multiple-regression equations in predicting systolic and diastolic blood pressures among all age groups. Bivariate Pearson correlation coefficients between body weight and systolic/diastolic blood pressures were .54/.48.

Diet: Salt Intake

Epidemiological studies have been used to assert that the prevalence of hypertension in populations is related to salt intake (Dahl & Love, 1957). While the populations studied (e.g., Polynesia, Micronesia, Africa) differ in many ways, salt intake has been consistently low in these societies. Animal and physiological studies have been used to support the hypothesis that sodium intake contributes to the determination of arterial pressure over a long period of time within the constraints imposed by an individual genetic endowment (Dahl, 1972).

In general, few topics have stimulated more controversial and inconsistent data than the hypothesis that salt intake elevates blood pressure

(Willett, 1981). Many have asserted that because salt intake in the United States is high (2.8 to 6.0 grams Na per day), greatly in excess of the 0.4 to 0.8 grams of sodium per day needed, a high prevalence of hypertension has resulted.

Studies elucidating the salt–hypertension hypothesis among children and adolescents have been sparse. Lanford et al. (1968) found higher blood pressures among rural than among city students, and inverse relationships between blood pressure and socioeconomic class. Langford & Watson (1973) selected 100 black female sibling pairs for study. Diastolic blood pressures were taken three times per day over eight days in the subjects' homes. Each of the girls also collected a urine specimen every 24 hours for six consecutive days. The Na/Ca ratio was lower ($x = 20.4$) among those with lower pressures (less than 105 mmHg systolic) than among those with higher pressures ($x = 34.4$; greater than 125 mmHg systolic). The ratio also was higher among rural females than among urban females ($x = 33.6$ versus 24.7, respectively). An inverse relationship also was found between socioeconomic status and Na/Ca excretion. However, blood pressures and sodium excretion of Na/Ca ratio were not correlated. An earlier study also failed to confirm correlations between sodium excretion or salt taste threshold and blood pressure (Langford & Watson, 1972). Salt may contribute to blood pressure, but not according to a direct linear function. Langford & Watson (1975) studied 108 black girls ages 19 to 21 using blood pressures collected over eight days and urine samples collected over six days. One significant correlation emerged: the correlation between diastolic blood pressure and Na/K ratio was .372. The authors concluded that, in the salt-sensitive portion of the population, blood pressure may be a direct function of salt intake and an indirect function of potassium and perhaps calcium intake.

Tuthill & Calabrese (1979) demonstrated a statistically significant upshift of 3 to 5 mmHg in mean blood pressure between high-school sophomores in two communities with water containing vastly different amounts of sodium. In a second study (Tuthill & Calabrese, 1981), they found identical results among third graders in the same two communities. A confounding factor in the second study was higher sodium intake in the community with higher-sodium water. Moreover, the data were supportive of the hypothesis of the sodium/blood-pressure relationships in the aggregate community level but not in the individual level. For these reasons, Willett (1981) suggested caution in accepting these promising results as definitive.

Data from the Bogalusa Heart Study suggest the hypothesis that a proportion of the population may be sensitive to salt (Berenson, Voors, Webber, Dalferes, & Harsha, 1979). Blacks with the highest blood pressures had lower levels than whites for similar 24-hour sodium levels. The black males of the high stratum showed a cluster of correlations pointing toward sensitivity of the sodium/potassium intake ratio. Blacks also have positive correlation between blood pressure and sodium intake (Frank, Farris, Mayor, Webber, & Berenson, 1981).

While the role of salt in the genesis and maintenance of elevated blood pressure among children and adolescents remains controversial, clinical studies among adults support the utility of reducing and controlling mild hypertension by restricting sodium intake (Corcoran, Taylor, & Page, 1951; Dole, Dahl, Cotzias, Eder, & Krebs, 1950). The relative potency of many antihypertensive medications parallels the potency of these drugs in promoting sustained sodium depletion. Finally, several recent clinical studies have supported the utility of reducing mild hypertension by restricting sodium intake. The Stanford 3-Community Study (Farquhar, Maccoby, Wood, Alexander, Breitrose, Brown, Hashell, McAlister, Meyer, Nash, & Stein 1977) also reported a significant longitudinal correlation between change in urinary sodium/potassium ratio and a change in blood pressure.

The Task Force on Blood Pressure Control (1977) concluded that the exact significance of salt intake in the genesis of hypertension has not been determined; however, there is general agreement that salt intake should be reduced by individuals with hypertension and by those at risk of developing it. The hypothesis that reduction of salt intake in children and adolescents will result in lower blood pressures remains to be determined.

Hemodynamics of Hypertension

The hemodynamics of hypertension have been studied extensively and reviewed recently by Frolich (1977). In some young subjects there appears to be an increased cardiac output and tachycardia indicating a hyperkinetic circulation. Such hyperkinetic or "high output types" also may be hypervolemic. Recent echocardiographic studies in children by Davignin, Rey, Payot, Biron, & Mongeau (1977) have confirmed prior invasive hemodynamic studies of others showing that hypertensive children can be either "hyperkinetic" or "hyperresistant."

Left ventricular hypertrophy characteristically is present at autopsy in patients with established hypertension. Recently, myocardial hypertrophy has been described in the spontaneously hypertensive rat before the appearance of elevated pressures and when hypertension is prevented by early immunosympathectomy (Cutilletta, Erinoff, Heller, Low, & Oparil, 1977; Cutilletta, Benjamin, Culpepper, & Oparil, 1978). These studies have suggested that myocardial hypertrophy may have a role in the pathogenesis of hypertension.

The echocardiogram has added a new dimension to the study of cardiovascular performance in hypertension (Sannerstedt, Bjure, & Varnaushas, 1970; Davignin et al., 1977). Measurements of stroke volume, systolic time intervals, and left ventricular wall thickness have shown subtle signs of diminished left ventricular function in some established hypertensives, but normal or increased cardiac performance in some young or borderline hypertensive subjects has shown them to be associated with faster heart rates and shorter preejection fractions and lower ratios of preejection period (PEP) and left ventricular ejection time (LVET).

Zahka, Neill, Kidd, Cutilletta, & Cutilletta (in press) examined 38 normotensive subjects of normotensive parents and 44 hypertensive subjects who were referred to a pediatric hypertension center. The average blood pressure of the hypertensive patients was $144 + 1.5/95 + 1.3$ mmHg, compared with $114 + 1.6/67 + 1.4$ mmHg ($p = 0.001$) in the normotensive group. While the difference is certainly significant, the elevated pressures would be considered to be only mildly elevated. Various indices of left ventricular mass, however, were significantly greater in the hypertensive patients compared with those of the normotensive controls. Eighty percent of the hypertensive patients met criteria of left ventricular hypertrophy. Furthermore, the degree of cardiac hypertrophy correlated poorly with either the systolic, diastolic, or mean blood pressures. A similar lack of correlation between hypertrophy and blood pressure has been reported in adult hypertensive patients. Left ventricular hypertrophy seems to persist despite good therapeutic control and is present even in borderline hypertension. It could be argued that a degree of hypertrophy could be expected in patients with pressure overload; however, it appears that the degree of hypertrophy found by Zahka et al. (in press) is out of proportion to the level of hypertension. Based upon the hypothesis, myocardial hypertrophy may be, at least in part, independent of the degree of hypertension and could have a role in the pathogenesis of the syndrome. The presence of hypertrophy, therefore, could prove useful in identifying patients who may go on to develop hypertension.

Behavioral Factors

It has been noted for some time that individuals differ in their pattern and degree of autonomic response to environmental stimulation (Lacey & Lacey, 1962). An early individual-difference variable correlated with exaggerated blood pressure response was the presence of cardiovascular disease. Malmo & Shagass (1949) reported that patients with cardiovascular problems reacted to stimulation with cardiovascular responses, while patients with head and neck aches responded with muscular responses.

Engel & Bickford (1961) found that patients with essential hypertension responded consistently to all stressful stimuli with increased systolic blood pressure, while normotensives did not.

There are some data to support the hypothesized risk-factor status of cardiovascular reactivity. Hines (1937) measured blood pressures of 400 normotensive children while they were subjected to a cold pressor test. The children were subdivided into "normal reactors" and "hyperreactors" (those whose pressures rose above 25/20 mmHg; 18% of the sample) on the basis of blood pressure increases during the test. Barnett, Hines, Schirger, & Gage (1963) followed 207 of the sample 27 years later. A significant proportion of the hyperreactors became hypertensive, while none of the normal reactors became hypertensive.

Two recent studies have assessed the relation of family variables to exaggerated blood pressure reactivity in adolescents. Falkner, Onesti, Angelakos, Fernandes, & Langman (1979) studied blood pressure response during mental arithmetic in adolescents with varying risk for developing essential hypertension. Three groups were studied: genetic hypertensives (N = 33) were those with normal basal blood pressure but at least one parent with essential hypertension; labile genetic hypertensives (N = 17) were those who already showed elevated basal blood pressure and also had at least one parent with essential hypertension; controls (N = 25) were those who had normal basal blood pressure and no family history of hypertension. [Based on recent studies and reconceptualizations, we would prefer the term "borderline" to the term "labile" used by those investigators; see Insel & Chadwick (in press) and Horan, Kennedy, & Padgett (1981)]. Subjects were male and female, black and white, ages 14 to 15 years. Labile genetic hypertensives and normotensive genetic subjects showed greater sustained increases than controls in systolic and diastolic blood pressure during mental arithmetic. Post-stress plasma catecholamines were higher in the labile and genetic hypertensives than in the control subjects. The investigators concluded that these findings demonstrated increased central nervous system adrenergic activity and cardiovascular responses in labile hypertensives and in normotensive subjects with a genetic risk for developing hypertension.

Baer, Vincent, Williams, Bourianoff, & Bartlett (1980) studied family interactions and posed some interesting questions regarding transmission of hypertension in families. Three-member families (father, mother, and boy or girl aged eight to 13 years) of hypertensive (N = 16) or normotensive (N = 15) fathers were videotaped as they interacted under standardized conditions calling for disagreement. Families with hypertensive fathers showed more negative interactions than families with normotensive fathers. Following these interactions, blood pressures of children in hypertensive families rose, whereas blood pressures in normotensive families fell. In the hypertensive families, there was a positive correlation between frequency of negative nonverbal parental behavior and postinterview systolic blood pressure ($r = .52$, $p < .05$).

Type A (coronary prone) Behavior. The so-called Type A behavior pattern has been associated repeatedly with increased acute blood pressure response to stress. This responsivity is one hypothesized pathway by which Type A might express itself in disease. According to Brand, Rosenman, Sholtz, & Friedman (1976), "Type A behavior is characterized by enhanced aggressiveness and competitive drive, preoccupation with deadlines, and chronic impatience and sense of time urgency in contrast to the more relaxed and less hurried Type B behavior pattern." The Western Collaborative Group study (Brand et al., 1976) and the Framingham study (Haynes, Feinleib, & Kannel, 1980) have both provided prospective verification that Type A is a risk factor for cardiovascular disease and that this effect is independent of such traditional risk factors as smoking, blood pressure, and cholesterol. Haynes, Feinleib, Levine, Scotch, & Kannel (1978) developed a 300-item questionnaire for use in the Framingham prospective study. The questionnaire contains 14 subscales (reliability from .64 to .86) in three general areas: (1) behavior types: Type A men, Type A women, emotional lability, ambitiousness, noneasygoing; (2)situational stress: nonsupport from boss, marital disagreement, marital dissatisfaction, aging worries, personal worries; (3) somatic strain: tension state, daily stress, anxiety symptoms, and anger symptoms. There was moderate to good (67% to 80%) concordance with the structured interview in discriminating Type A from Type B subjects.

In a cross-sectional study of 1822 persons 45 to 77 years of age, Haynes et al. (1978) found that women (45 to 64 years of age) with coronary heart disease (CHD) scored significantly higher on Type A, emotional lability, aging worries, tension, and anger symptom scales than did women free of CHD. Among men under 65, Type A, aging worries, daily stress, and tension were associated with prevalence of myocardial infarction.

Haynes et al. (1980) followed 1674 subjects in the Framingham study for eight years. Women who developed CHD scored significantly higher in Framingham Type A, suppressed hostility, tension, and anger than did women remaining free of CHD. The prospective study demonstrates the utility of the Framingham Type A scale in predicting disease.

Type A behavior also has been related to the incidence and prevalence of clinical CHD in men and women (Haynes et al., 1980), angiographically determined severity of atherosclerosis (Blumenthal, Williams, Kong, et al., 1978; Friedman, Rosenman, Straus, et al., 1968), and the progression of atherosclerosis in men (Krantz, Schaeffer, Daria, Dembroski, & MacDougall, in press).

Type A Behavior and Reactivity in Children. The relationship between Type A behavior and blood pressure reactivity in children and adolescents has been documented in recent research. Siegel & Leitch (1981) found a positive correlation between elevated systolic blood pressure and Type A behavior in adolescents. Children and adolescents in the Bogalusa Heart Study who reported that they felt an exaggerated sense of time urgency had higher mean arterial blood pressure than students who responded negatively to this item (Voors, Sklor, Hunter, & Berenson, 1982). Spiga & Petersen (1981) studied fourth- and fifth-grade children in a Catholic school. The Mathews Youth Test for Health (MYTH) was used; the 18 highest- and 18 lowest-scoring males were selected to participate. These students were matched in dyads by Type A and B behaviors so that there were six AA, six AB, and six BB dyads. The dyads played a mixed-motive game in which each player could choose to compete or cooperate on each trial; rewards for individual players were contingent upon both players' choices. Type A's in AA dyads showed more competitiveness than Type A's in AB dyads and Type B's in BB dyads. Type A's in AA dyads also exhibited greater fluctuations in blood pressure during the task than other subjects.

A Multivariate Look

In this author's laboratory research, an effort has been made to examine in combination the relative contribution of family history, ponderosity, age, and the Type A behavior pattern to basal blood pressure and to blood pressure response in adolescents. Subjects (21 black and 21 white males ranging in age from 14 to 17 years) were recruited from the Pediatric Blood Pressure Center at The Johns Hopkins Hospital and from local high schools. The characteristics of the subjects are presented in Table 4.1.

Subjects were enrolled in the study after at least three two-successive blood pressure determinations using suitable cuff sizes had established their basal blood pressure. Approximately one week after the third clinic-based assessment, subjects returned to the Small Group Programmed Environment Laboratory at the Phipps Psychiatric Clinic at The Johns Hopkins Hospital.

Each subject was escorted to the recreation area, where he was seated at a desk. An interview took place to collect additional data on family history. The subject was weighed and height was measured. The subject then completed two measures of Type A behavior, the Jenkins Activity Survey (JAS) adapted for adolescents, and the Bortner Rating Scale. The adult version of the JAS is a self-administered questionnaire (60 items) with "Type A," "Hard-Driving," "Speed and Impatience," and "Job Involvement" subscales (Dembroski & MacDougall, 1978). Spiga & Petersen

Table 4.1
Participants in the Study of Blood Pressure Reactivity ($n = 42$)

	Mean	S.D.
Age	15.60	1.40
Weight (lbs.)	153.00	28.50
Average percent above ideal weight	1.10	0.22
Systolic blood pressure (resting)	122.80	11.60
Diastolic blood pressure (resting)	64.20	13.40
Heart rate (resting)	70.00	9.80
Type A (Jenkins)[1]	−2.19	8.33
Job involvement (Jenkins)[1]	−8.83	8.80
Speed and impatience (Jenkins)[1]	−3.54	8.89
Hard-driving and competitive (Jenkins)[1]	−8.30	14.24
Bortner Rating Scale	165.34	34.32
Percent with hypertensive parents	54	
Points on Alluisi Task during 15 minutes on CRT	78.46	22.58

[1]These are standard scores, normalized on a version of the Jenkins Activity Survey developed for adolescents (Spiga & Petersen, 1981).

(1981) adapted a shortened form (47 items) of this instrument for adolescents, and the adapted version was used in our study.

Following completion of the written tests, the subject was escorted into the small workshop area, where he was seated before the cathode-ray terminal (CRT). He was instructed about the sequence of events to follow and was fitted with a remotely monitored and controlled blood pressure cuff (Vita Stat Model 900-5), a digital thermistor for monitoring skin temperature, and an optically transduced plethysmograph for monitoring peripheral blood flow. Each subject was instructed in how to complete the Alluisi Performance Battery and was given 15 minutes of adaptation to the room and to the monitoring devices. Each subject then was exposed to alternating 15 minute periods of (1) baseline, quiet resting; (2) task performance on the Alluisi Performance Battery on the CRT; (3) baseline, quiet rest; and (4) metronome conditioned relaxation.

The Alluisi Performance Battery requires subjects to complete five tasks simultaneously: probability monitoring, horizontal addition and subtraction of 3-digit numbers, matching to sample histograms, detecting when a stationary signal moves, and detecting when a moving signal becomes stationary (Emurian, Emurian, & Brady, 1978).

Stepwise multiple-regression equations with free entry of variables were computed to assess independent variables related to basal blood pressure and to blood pressure change from baseline to Alluisi. The number of variables permitted to enter each equation was limited to five so that models would not be overdetermined. Tables 4.2 and 4.3 present multiple-regression results showing predictors of baseline systolic and diastolic blood pressure. Our findings were similar to those from the Bogalusa Heart Study (Berenson, 1980) in that we were able to account for 40 percent of the variance in systolic blood pressure. Ponderosity, age, and parental hypertension were significant predictor variables. Most important, measures of Type A behavior entered into the multiple-regression equations and added significantly to the prediction.

We were able to account for 51 percent of the variance in baseline diastolic blood pressure using both ponderosity and Type A behavior as independent variables. This may represent one of the strongest documentations in adolescents of the relation between behavioral factors and baseline blood pressures; certainly it deserves replication.

We were primarily interested in accounting for blood pressure response during performance on the Alluisi Task. Tables 4.4, 4.5, and 4.6 present multiple-regression results showing predictors of the absolute and relative (percent increase above baseline) changes from baseline to Alluisi in systo-

Table 4.2
Dependent Variable: Baseline Systolic Blood Pressure

Independent Variable	Beta	R
Weight/height^2	.410	.47
Age	.228	.55
Parental hypertension	.298	.58
Job involvement (JAS)	.212	.62
Type A (Bortner)	.149	.64

$R^2 = .41$
$F = 4.62 \ (p < .01)$

Table 4.3
Dependent Variable: Baseline Diastolic Blood Pressure

Independent Variable	Beta	R
Weight/height^2	.608	.56
Type A (Bortner)	.286	.64
Hard-driving (JAS)	.307	.67
Age	.275	.69
Type A (JAS)	−.295	.71

$R^2 = .50$
$F = 7.05 \ (p < .001)$

Table 4.4
Dependent Variable: Absolute Change in Systolic Blood Pressure

Independent Variable	Beta	B
Alluisi points	−.442	.38
Bortner Type A	.239	.48
Mean baseline systolic pressure	.195	.54
Parental hypertension	−.273	.58

$R^2 = .34$
$F = 4.57 \, (p < .01)$

Table 4.5
Dependent Variable: Relative Change in Systolic Blood Pressure

Independent Variable	Beta	B
Bortner Type A	.372	.366
Alluisi points	−.404	.531
Weight/height^2	.254	.575
Parental hypertension	−.214	.606
Age	.078	.617

$R^2 = .381$
$F = 4.06 \, (p < .01)$

Table 4.6
Dependent Variable: Relative Change in Diastolic Blood Pressure

Independent Variable	Beta	R
Weight/height^2	−.294	.32
Age	.161	.38
Race	.093	.39

$R^2 = .16$
$F = 3.62 \, (p < .05)$

lic and diastolic blood pressure. Behavioral factors entered most strongly in predicting absolute and relative systolic blood pressure change. Performance on the Alluisi task was negatively related to systolic blood pressure increases (that is, students who performed better showed smaller relative and absolute increases in systolic pressure), and performance was positively related to Type A as measured by the Bortner inventory. Baseline systolic pressure, parental hypertension, and relative obesity were other variables entering into these equations.

Significant Research Needs

Type A Behavior and Reactivity

Type A behavior is a relatively poor predictor of coronary heart disease (CHD). Although the adjusted risk ratio in the Western Collaborative Group Study was 1.87 (Brand et al., 1976), only about 10 percent of men diagnosed as Type A developed early clinical signs of coronary heart disease. Type A behavior also is a relatively poor predictor of cardiovascular reactivity. Work in several laboratories has demonstrated that Type A college students and working adults show greater average cardiovascular reactivity to a variety of performance challenges than do their Type B peers. In any sample, Type A's will on the average show greater overall increases in blood pressure and heart rate when presented with challenging tasks under ego-involving conditions. Type A relates only imperfectly to cardiovascular reactivity. Between-subject variability within types is quite high.

Some promising data have been collected relating components of Type A to cardiovascular disease. Matthews, Glass, Rosenman, & Bortner (1977) showed that speed of activity, achievement, and job involvement were not related to CHD. Potential for hostility, competitiveness, impatience, irritability, and vigorous voice stylistics were related to overt manifestations of CHD. Jenkins, Zyzanski, & Rosenman (1976) reported that sense of time urgency, job promotions, and past achievements were most characteristic of those manifesting silent myocardial infarction. The next step in this research should involve relating the components of Type A behavior to exaggerated cardiovascular reactivity.

Type A Behavior and
Natural-Environment Reactivity

The evidence relating Type A behavior to blood pressure response in the natural environment is mixed. Manuck, Corse, & Winkelman (1979) and Waldron, Hickey, McPherson, Butensky, Gruss, Overall, Schmade, & Wohlmuth (1980) provided some evidence that the Jenkins Activity Scale defined Type A working adults and college students as showing higher blood pressure levels during their daily activities than Type B adults and students. DeBacker, Kornitzer, Kittel, et al. (1979) found no differences in catecholamine excretion, heart rate, or ECG abnormalities between Type A and Type B factory workers in Belgium.

Other Variables Influencing
Natural-Environment Reactivity

To our knowledge there are no published data concerning the degree to which laboratory measures of cardiovascular reactivity are correlated with similar measures obtained in daily life. The assumption is made that laboratory assessments are representative of reactivity in the natural environment. The hypothesis that the two are related is reasonable, but empirical study of the degree of relationship clearly is needed.

Blood pressure varies with sleep, physical activity, and emotional stimulation; this has been recognized for many years (Brash & Fairweather, 1901; Addis, 1922). Average variations of 36 mmHg (in normotensives) and 55 mmHg (in hypertensives) were observed during the day by Mueller & Brown (1930). Continuous recordings of direct arterial pressure have confirmed the importance of sleep and physical activity in determining blood pressure (Bevan, Honour, & Stott, 1969; Littler, West, Honour, & Sleight, 1978). The short-term changes during smoking (Cellina, Honour, & Littler, 1975), defecating (Littler, Honour, & Sleight, 1974) and coitus (Bevan et al., 1969) have been documented amply.

Significant changes in blood pressures can be produced by a great variety of stimuli in the laboratory; however, the extent to which normal environmental and psychological influences cause variation in blood pressure in the course of an individual's everyday life has received relatively little study. In his provocative monograph, Pickering (1961) states:

> If the provisional hypothesis is entertained that long continued and oft repeated emotional rises in pressure eventually raise pressure more continuously, then the mind may be envisaged as a major factor in the pathogenesis of hypertension. Factors that operate through the mind may be of importance, but they have so far neither been identified or measured. In fact, the identification and measurement of the influence of the environment in determining arterial pressure is the most important field to be explored if we wish to know precisely the factors concerned in the etiology of essential hypertension.

Lack of data about human cardiovascular function under natural circumstances retards better understanding of the conjectured relationships between adaptational responses to environmental forces and the development of cardiovascular disease.

Sokolow and his colleagues at the Cardiovascular Research Institute at the University of California, San Francisco, have been in the forefront in studying variations in blood pressure by means of ambulatory monitoring.

They found that ambulatory blood pressures were lower than office blood pressures in 80 percent of patients studied (Sokolow, Werdegar, Kain, & Hinman, 1966). Target-organ damage was associated more closely with ambulatory than with office blood pressures, and this has been noted in patients whose blood pressure is presumably under control with antihypertensive medications (Perloff & Sokolow, 1978).

Sokolow, Werdegar, Perloff, Cowan, & Berenstuhl (1970) reported an initial attempt to relate daily life events to blood pressure variation during the day in 50 adult patients with essential hypertension. To our knowledge, this is the only published study attempting to relate variations in mood to variations in blood pressure. Subjects wore the Remler semiautomated blood pressure monitor. They were instructed to inflate the cuff themselves every 30 minutes throughout the day. Subjects also kept a logbook in which they noted activities and events in the day that coincided with blood pressure measurements. The logbook also contained a checklist of adjectives on which subjects rated themselves at each blood pressure measurement. Obviously, any system that requires the subject to stop and inflate a blood pressure cuff would influence both mood and blood pressure. Moreover, subjects might not take their blood pressure during times of increased emotional intensity.

Of interest to this discussion is the utility of self-ratings to discriminate variability in blood pressure across the day. Ratings of alertness, anxiety, and time pressure (note the similarity to components of Type A) discriminated the highest from the lowest systolic and diastolic blood pressure readings. Significant intra-individual correlations were found between systolic and diastolic blood pressure and anxiety, time pressure, negative affect (positive correlation) and contentment (negative correlation).

Three research needs emerge from this analysis.

1. *Multivariate studies are needed to sort out the contributions of individual variables and their interactions.* One important outcome of the search for etiological factors in cardiovascular disease has been the realization that the disease results from a complex interplay of constitutional, environmental, and behavioral factors. Research in reactivity has been especially deficient, however, because single (e.g., Type A behavior, family history) variables have been studied in isolation.

2. *We need to identify components of Type A behavior related to the development of cardiovascular disease and to exaggerated blood pressure reactivity to environmental stressors.* The specificity value of a global rating of Type A is quite low. The majority of adult males in a variety of subpopulations in the United States has been found to show the Type A

behavior pattern. Only a small subset of these Type A persons develops cardiovascular disease at an early age. The specificity value of Type A in predicting cardiovascular reactivity is also quite low. Type A's, on the average, show greater blood pressure response than Type B's in socially challenging and competitive situations; however, not all Type A's show the exaggerated response.

3. *We need more data concerning the degree to which laboratory measures of cardiovascular reactivity predict reactivity in everyday life. Also, we need better and more definitive data relating global assessments of Type A and reactivity in everyday life.* Rosenman, Brand, Sholtz, & Friedman (1976) found differences between extreme Type A's and B's in catecholamine production during the workday. Manuck et al. (1979) and Waldron et al. (1980) showed that Type A adults and college students manifested higher blood pressure levels than Type B's during their daily activities. However, differences in blood pressure were found between A and B air-traffic controllers (Cobb & Rose, 1973). A and B factory workers in Belgium showed no differences in catecholamine excretion, heart rate, or ECG abnormalities during their workday (DeBacker et al., 1979).

Treating Elevated Blood Pressure

Medication Management

There is as yet no consensus on the most appropriate course of medical management of juvenile hypertension. Children and adolescents with borderline or mild elevations in blood pressure typically do not require medication (Sinaiko & Mirkin, 1978). In these cases, the Task Force on Blood Pressure Control (1977) recommends annual reevaluation, counseling on weight control and salt intake, and encouragement to be active physically. Antihypertensive drug therapy is recommended in individuals with persistent elevations in diastolic blood pressure above 90 mmHg if they are between seven and 12 years of age and in certain individuals between 13 and 18 years of age. Medication is recommended for elevations above 100 mmHg for all individuals from seven to 18 years of age.

Medication regimens are implemented in a "stepped-care" approach. Thiazide diuretics usually are selected first. The antihypertensive effects are related to decreases in plasma volume and extracellular fluid. The only known side-effect of thiazide therapy in children is decrease in serum potassium, which is treated with potassium supplements.

If the child's blood pressure does not respond to thiazide, then a beta-blocking agent or methyldopa is recommended as a supplement to thiazide. The mechanism of action of beta-blocking agents in lowering blood pressure is poorly understood. Suppression of the renin-angiotension system and action on beta adrenergic receptors located in blood pressure regulatory mechanisms in the brain have been proposed (Sinaiko & Mirkin, 1978). These agents should not be used if asthma is diagnosed; moreover, bradycardia is an infrequent complication of therapy.

Methyldopa competes with dopa in the synthesis of norepinephrine, so stores of norepinephrine can become depleted. However, it is thought that methyldopa acts on the central vasomotor control center in lowering blood pressure (Day & Roach, 1974). Side-effects include sedation, hepatitis, and hemolysis.

If this course is ineffective, then a vasodilator such as hydralizine is usually added to the regimen. Vasodilators act by reducing vascular wall tension (Sinaiko & Mirkin, 1978). The high incidence of side-effects limit their usefulness. Regularly seen are headache, flushness, tachycardia, salt and water retention, and increased cardiac output.

It is also possible that aggressive antihypertensive therapy will not lower the juvenile's blood pressure to an acceptable level so hospitalization may be required.

Important issues related to antihypertensive drug therapy are the potential effects on the central nervous system. Long-term deleterious effects on the development of various organs and systems also must be evaluated to validate the continued use of these medications. Of more immediate concern to the physician is the predicted high rate of nonadherence to medical regimens that potentially can undermine therapy.

Weight Loss

Weight loss can promote blood pressure reduction among adults (Tyroler, Heyden, et al., 1975; Chiang, Perlman, & Epstein, 1969). It has been suggested, however, that drops in blood pressure with weight loss are due entirely to the concomitant reduction in salt intake (Dahl, 1972). Reisin, Abel, Modau, Silverberg, Eliahon, & Modan (1978), however, reported reductions in blood pressure concomitant with weight loss and independent of restriction in salt intake among adults. Patients, overweight and hypertensive, fell into three groups: those not receiving antihypertensive drug therapy (Group 1) and those on regular drug therapy but with inadequate control of hypertension (Groups 2a and 2b). Groups 1 and 2a received dietary counseling for weight loss, while Group 2b did not. All patients in Groups 1 and 2a lost at least 3 kg.; mean losses were 13.5 kg. (+6.3), and standard deviation was 14.9 (+5.3 kg.) during the same period. Seventy-five percent of Group 1 and 61 percent of Group 2a returned to a normal blood pressure, and correlations between weight loss and reductions in systolic and diastolic blood pressure were significant in both groups (Group 1 = .42/.56; Group 2a = .24/.30). Mean urinary sodium excretion from a 24-hour sample was similar following treatment among all three groups.

Coates et al., (1982) examined the relationships between weight loss and changes in blood pressures among normotensive but overweight adolescents. Subjects were 36 adolescents participating in a study of the efficacy of various treatment variables to facilitate weight loss. Prior to their participation in weight-loss classes, subjects reported to the laboratory on two separate mornings. After the subjects had been seated in the laboratory for several minutes, blood pressure was measured in the right arm using a standard sphygmomanometer. The subject was then left alone for 5 minutes, at which time the nurse returned to take a second reading. The same procedure was followed 24 weeks later following the end of the subjects' participation in the weight-loss classes.

Table 4.7 presents pre- and posttreatment values for weight and blood

Table 4.7
Changes in Weight and Blood Pressure during Weight Loss

	Pre	Post	Change
Weight	X = 179.06	169.98	−9.08**
	S.D. = 41.06	40.37	
	R = 136–269	122–182	
Percent overweight	X = 40.62	33.78	−6.84**
	S.D. = 23.13	24.74	
	R = 9–100	2.5–110	
Systolic blood pressure	X = 114.54	107.30	−7.25*
	S.D. = 10.34	14.28	
	R = 98–131	80–129	
Diastolic blood pressure	X = 72.84	66.27	−6.57**
	S.D. = 8.21	9.27	
	R = 75–93	51–85	

$*p < .05$
$** p < .01$

Adapted from T. J. Coates, R. W. Jeffery, L. A. Slinkard, J. D. Killen, & B. G. Danaher. Frequency of contact and monetary reward in weight loss, lipid change, and blood pressure reduction with adolescents. *Behavior Therapy*, 1982, *13*(2), 175–185.

pressure for all subjects. Blood pressures reported represent the average of the second reading taken at each of two assessment sessions. Pre- and posttreatment values were compared using the *t*-tests for paired samples.

Relaxation and Biofeedback

A collaborative effort among the Division of Pediatric Cardiology, the Division of Behavioral Biology, and the Division of Health Education at The Johns Hopkins Medical Institution is in progress. Three interventions are being evaluated: medical management, health education, and biofeedback/relaxation.

Anderson & Masek (1980) reported an initial study of health education involving a psychophysiological training in which 27 adolescents, ages 12 to 18, were referred from The Johns Hopkins Pediatric Blood Pressure Center. Eligibility for inclusion in the study was based on clinic observations of systolic or diastolic pressure levels above the 90th percentile for sex and age using the norms from the Task Force on Blood Pressure Control (1977). The experimental design of the treatment program called for six biweekly visits over a three-month period. The treatment program included (1) training and practice in Bensonian meditation; (2) training and practice in self-monitoring of blood pressure; and (3) health education to reduce salt intake.

Anderson & Masek's (1980) sequence of procedures in each clinic session, together with the timing of each blood pressure observation is paraphrased as follows:

1. Enter consulting room: experimenter and subject take concurrent ausculatory pressures.
2. Collect data sheets on home pressure and diet data.
3. Meditation room: attach physiological sensors.
4. Baseline monitoring period: three automatic pressure measurements over a ten-minute period.
5. Meditation period: two automatic pressure measurements over a ten-minute period.
6. Postmeditation period: one automatic pressure measurement over a five-minute period.
7. Detach physiological sensors.
8. Return to consulting room: experimenter and subject take concurrent pressures within five minutes.
9. Discuss home data and complete salt education procedures.
10. Final concurrent blood pressure measurement by subject and experimenter.

11. Subject is weighed.
12. Next appointment is set.

Each subject's blood pressures were recorded using three methods:

1. A Dinamap blood pressure recorder automatically monitored blood pressure every 5 minutes during meditation training.
2. Blood pressure was monitored both by the experimenter and by the subject, using an auscultatory procedure in the clinic consulting room.
3. The subject recorded his/her own blood pressure at home, also by the auscultatory method. Subjects recorded their blood pressure at home twice per day, once in the morning and once in the evening.

The experimenter's blood pressure monitoring accuracy was established and maintained by periodic reliability checks with two other project investigators. The accuracy of the subjects' pressure measurements was established and maintained by weekly concurrent observations with the experimenter.

The double-headed-stethoscope technique was used for concurrent blood pressure observations. Mean differences between the experimenter's and the subjects' blood pressure recordings averaged $-0.92 + 2.8$ mmHg systolic and $0.054 + 1.4$ mmHg diastolic. The home data were discarded only if successive readings showed excessive variability. Two of the 14 subjects provided either an inadequate amount of data or readings of too questionable a validity to be used.

The subjects in the control group were seen twice in the clinic; once at the initial intake examination and again after a three-month interval. On each occasion three blood pressure readings were obtained by the same experimenter.

Table 4.8 presents baseline blood pressure levels and changes at three months for the treatment and control subjects using blood pressure measures obtained in the clinic. The data show that systolic ($t = 1.33$) and diastolic ($t = 0.10$) pressures were not significantly different at baseline. An analysis of covariance with baseline blood pressures as the covariate was used to compare posttreatment blood pressures of treatment and control subjects. Posttreatment systolic blood pressures of treatment subjects were significantly different from posttreatment systolic blood pressures of controls. Differences in posttreatment diastolic blood pressure were not significant.

These initial data are promising, but much work remains to be done before assertions about the efficacy of these procedures can be claimed definitively. Significant research questions and issues include (1) demon-

Table 4.8
Clinic Blood Pressures for Treatment and Control Subjects at Baseline and
Three Months Later

	Baseline: Mean (S.E.)	3 Months Later: Mean (S.E.)	Change from Baseline to 3 Months Later: Mean (S.E.)	F
Systolic				
Treatment (N = 14)	140.4 (3.80)	128.6 (3.02)	–11.7 (3.40)	5.514 (p = .027)*
Controls (N = 13)	146.0 (1.82)	141.7 (3.61)	– 4.3 (2.65)	
Diastolic				
Treatment (N = 14)	86.0 (2.80)	79.6 (3.22)	– 6.4 (2.60)	1.729 (p = .201)**
Controls (N = 13)	86.4 (3.47)	83.1 (2.25)	– 2.08 (2.80)	

*F–Ratio, analysis of covariance comparing posttreatment, systolic blood pressure using baseline blood pressure as the covariate = 5.514, $p = .027$, $df = 1/24$.
**F–Ratio, analysis of covariance comparing posttreatment diastolic blood pressure using baseline blood pressure as the covariate = 1.729, $p = .201$, $df = 1/24$.
Adapted from D. E. Anderson & B. Masek. Bensonian meditation in the treatment of adolescent hypertension. Paper presented at the meetings of the Society for Behavioral Medicine, New York, 1980.

stration of efficacy of relaxation in lowering blood pressure over a long period of time; (2) studies of efficacy of relaxation in relation to placebo controls; (3) demonstration of effects using 24-hour ambulatory monitoring to obtain estimates of the generality of effects; and (4) studies of the ability of relaxation and other health education strategies in altering the natural history of blood pressure.

Stress-Management Training

The stress-management program views responses to stress-provoking situations as being learned responses that can be replaced by newly learned and more adaptive responses. When the person faces a stressful situation, the autonomic nervous system is aroused. The cardiovascular system, for example, may indicate stress by an increase in heart rate, pulse rate, and blood pressure. The cognitive component of stress is characterized by intrusive thoughts and images, racing thoughts, worries, and by difficulty in controlling or focusing attention. The behavioral component of stress is characterized by increased rate in kinds of motoric activity (face scratching, eye blinks, pacing) and by polyphasic activity. The program attempts to teach the subjects to become aware and identify stress in their daily lives, to become aware of the specific ways in which they experience tension, and to learn strategies for reducing their stress.

An overview of the stress-management protocol is presented in Table 4.9. This program is built upon a similar strategy developed for classroom teachers by Guzicki & Coates (1979). In the first session, the subject is introduced to the training program and the conceptualization of stress and is taught to discriminate those situations causing personal stress and tension. Stress and tension as discrete responses are introduced first when the therapist discusses personal examples of situations causing stress together with the reactions she or he has experienced. Following this, the subject is encouraged to discuss situations relevant to him or her and is assisted in describing personal reactions of stress and tension. Checklists for identify-

Table 4.9
Stress-Management Protocol

Session #1	Definitions of stress; components of stress
	Discussion of situations in which stress is commonly experienced; how stress interferes with the ability to act productively
	Progressive Relaxation Training #1
Between Sessions	Practice relaxation once per day
	Record practice times on forms
	Note stressful situations and reactions
Session #2	Feedback on Progressive Relaxation
	Continuation of discussion of stressful situations and reactions
	Progressive Relaxation Training #2
Between Sessions	Continue practice each day
	Continue to note practice times on forms
Session #3	Feedback on Progressive Relaxation
	Introduction to cue-controlled relaxation, practice
	Role-play using cue-controlled relaxation in a specific stress-provoking situation
Between Sessions	Continue practicing Progressive Relaxation
	Practice cue-controlled relaxation alone and try out in one prerehearsed situation
Session #4	Discussion of results with cue-controlled relaxation
	Role-play using cue-controlled relaxation in other situations identified as stress-provoking
Assignment	Continue using Progressive Relaxation and cue-controlled relaxation
	Further sessions devoted to this area as needed

Adapted from J. Guzicki & T. J. Coates. Cue-controlled relaxation for the classroom teacher. *Journal of School Psychology*, 1979, *18*, 17–24.

ing stress reactions and stressful situations are used to aid this process. This is followed by training in progressive relaxation (cf. Bernstein & Borkovec, 1973; Coates & Thoresen, 1977). The exercise is taped to facilitate home practice. Subjects are asked to practice relaxation once per day and to record on self-monitoring forms times at which they practice relaxation. They also are asked to note and write down specific situations during the week in which they noticed that they experienced stress of a moderate or severe degree.

The second session introduces no new material but involves continued discussion of situations causing stress and indicators of stress. Role-playing is used to help subjects identify personal stress reactions. Progressive relaxation is practiced a second time. The third session introduces the subject to cue-controlled relaxation. While relaxed, each subject is asked to attend to her or his breathing and to repeat the cue word "Relax" subvocally with each exhalation. The therapist then repeats the word in synchrony with the subject's exhalation five times, and the subject continues aloud for 15 more pairings. The subject then practices cue-controlled relaxation in simulated anxiety-provoking situations. The therapist first models feeling stress and using cue-controlled relaxation to reduce it. The subject then is encouraged to role-play cue-controlled relaxation in situations identified earlier as stress provoking. Between sessions, the subject is encouraged to practice cue-controlled relaxation alone and to try it out in one prerehearsed situation.

During the final session, progress and problems are discussed. Other stress-provoking situations are identified and the subject and therapist rehearse methods for managing stress during these situations. Feedback and further practice are conducted as needed in subsequent sessions.

Data evaluating the program are quite preliminary, but an example from one case study illustrates the techniques and outcomes. The patient was a 14-year-old black male whose blood pressures were consistently above the 90th percentile using the norms from the Task Force on Pediatric Blood Pressure (see Figure 4.3). He was referred to us from the Pediatric Primary Clinic for complaints of headache, dizziness, nosebleeds, and school absenteeism. He was living with his maternal grandmother after his mother asked him to leave her home when she began living with a woman in a love relationship. The grandmother's home was located in a ghetto section of Baltimore, and the patient reported many fights and other altercations on the streets and at school. He cited this as a major reason for refusing to go to school.

Treatment in stress management revolved around the stresses of visiting his mother and his embarrassment at her homosexual affair, dealing with his grandmother over unreasonable demands, and dealing with the stres-

Figure 4.3 Average Blood Pressures. Taken at baseline (weeks 1–3), during treatment (weeks 4–7), and at follow-up (week 16). Each blood pressure represents the average of 3 blood pressures taken after 10 minutes' rest and taken 5 minutes apart. Open symbols represent averages from 24-hour blood pressures.

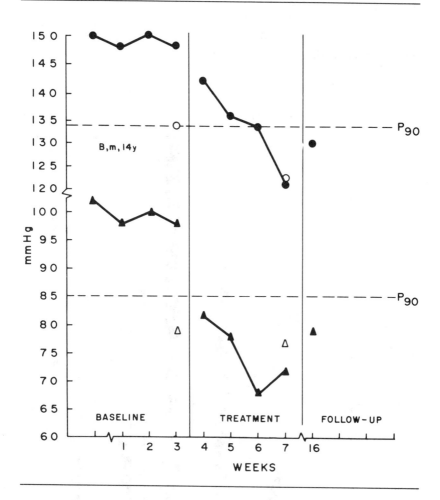

ses of school work and harrassment from other students. Training in progressive relaxation and the stress-management training were associated with blood pressure lowering, and this persisted at follow-up 16 weeks after the start of treatment.

We also obtained blood pressures over a 24-hour period every 7.5

minutes using automated blood pressure techniques (Horan et al., 1981).
The patient wore the automated cuff for the 24-hour period, and blood
pressures were taken and recorded automatically using the Del Mar
Avionics automated blood pressure monitor. Figures 4.4 and 4.5 present
the percentages of systolic and diastolic blood pressure at each level for one
day before and one day following treatment. Examination of the average

Figure 4.4   Systolic Blood Pressures. Taken every 7.5 minutes over 24
hours during baseline (week 3) and during week 7 of treatment.

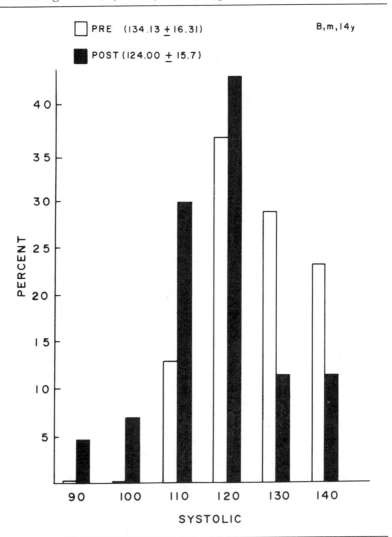

Figure 4.5 Diastolic Blood Pressures. Taken every 7.5 minutes over 24 hours during baseline (week 3) and during week 7 of treatment.

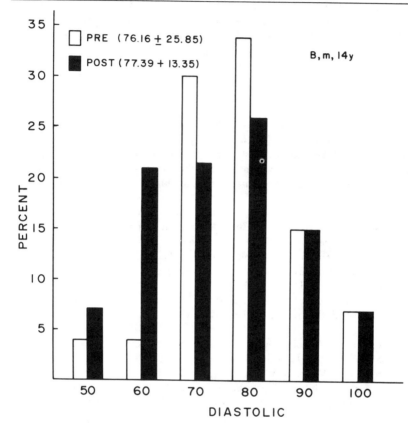

blood pressures obtained from the 24-hour recording shows that mean systolic pressure was reduced about 10 mmHg from 134.13 to 124.00 mmHg. Diastolic pressure did not reduce, but there was a considerable reduction in the standard deviation of the diastolic pressure, indicating a reduction in variability. Examination of the histograms indicates a shifting of the distribution of blood pressures toward the lower end of the scale.

A Final Comment

A careful reading of this chapter reveals that the field of adolescent blood pressure study is lopsided. We know quite a bit about how to measure blood pressure and about the correlates of basal blood pressure in pediatric populations. There are some descriptive data on blood pressure responsivity. Beyond that, the data are scanty. The significance of blood pressure responsivity and methods for modifying it have not been identified, and much work remains to be done in lowering basal blood pressure among adolescents. The ultimate health significance of these measures remains to be established in longitudinal studies.

References

Addis, T. Blood pressure and pulse rate levels under basal and daytime conditions. *Archives of Internal Medicine*, 1922, *39*, 539.

American Heart Association. *Heart facts.* Dallas, Tex.: Aita, 1976.

Anderson, D. E., & Masek, B. Bensonian meditation in the treatment of adolescent hypertension. Paper presented at the meetings of the Society for Behavioral Medicine, New York, 1980.

Baer, P. E., Vincent, J. P., Williams, B. J., Bourianoff, C. G., & Bartlett, P. C. Behavioral response to induced conflict in families with a hypertensive father. *Hypertension*, 1980, *2:42*, 70–77.

Barnett, P. H., Hines, E. A., Schirger, A., & Gage, R. P. Blood pressure and vascular reactivity to the cold pressor test. *Journal of the American Medical Association*, 1963, *183*, 845–848.

Beaglehole, R., Salmond, C. E., & Prior, I. A. M. Blood pressure studies in Polynesian children. In O. Paul (ed.), *Epidemiology and control of hypertension.* New York: Grune & Stratton, 1975, 407–419.

Berenson, G. S. *Cardiovascular risk factors in children: The Bogalusa Heart Study.* New York: Oxford University Press, 1980.

Berenson, G. S., Voors, A. W., Webber, L. S., Dalferes, E. R., & Harsha, D. W. Racial differences of parameters associated with blood pressure levels in children. The Bogalusa Heart Study. *Metabolism*, 1979, *28:12*, 1218–1228.

Bernstein, D. A., & Borkovec, T. D. *Progressive relaxation training.* Champaign, Ill.: Research Press, 1973.

Bevan, A. T., Honour A. J., & Stott, F. H. Direct arterial pressure recording in unrestricted man. *Clinical Science*, 1969, *36*, 329.

Blumenthal, J. A., Williams, R. B., Kong, Y., et al. Type A behavior pattern and coronary atherosclerosis. *Circulation*, 1978, *58:4*, 634–639.

Brand, R. J., Rosenman, R. H., Sholtz, R. I., and Friedman, M. Multivariate prediction of coronary heart disease in the Western Collaborative Group Study compared to the findings of the Framingham study. *Circulation*, 1976, *53*, 348–355.

Brash, L. E., & Fairweather, R. Observations on changes in blood pressure during normal sleep. *American Journal of Physiology*, 1901, *5*, 199–210.

Cellina, F. U., Honour, A. J., & Littler, W. A. Direct arterial pressure, heart rate, and electrocardiogram during cigarette smoking in unrestricted patients. *American Heart Journal*, 1975, *89:1*, 18–25.

Chenoweth, A. D. High blood pressure: A national concern. *Journal of School Health,* 1973, 43, 307–308.

Chiang, B. N., Perlman, L. V., & Epstein, F. H. Overweight and hypertension: A review. *Circulation,* 1969, *39,* 403–421.

Coates, T. J., Jeffery, R. W., Slinkard, L. A., Killen, J. D., & Danaher, B. G. Frequency of contact and monetary reward in weight loss, lipid change, and blood pressure reduction with adolescents. *Behavior Therapy,* 1982, *13*(2), 175–185.

Coates, T. J., Parker, F. C., & Kolodner, K. Stress and heart disease: Does blood pressure reactivity offer a link? In T. J. Coates, A. C. Peterson, & C. Perry (eds.), *Adolescent health: Crossing the barriers.* New York: Academic Press, in press.

Coates, T. J., & Thoresen, C. E. *How to sleep better.* Englewood Cliffs, N. J.: Prentice-Hall, 1977.

Coates, T. J., & Thoresen, C. E. Using generalizability theory in behavioral observations. *Behavior Therapy,* 1978, *9,* 605–613.

Cobb, S., & Rose, R. M. Hypertension, peptic ulcer, and diabetes in air traffic controllers. *Journal of the American Medical Association,* 1973, *224,* 489–492.

Comstock, G. W. An epidemiologic study of blood pressure levels in a biracial community in the southern United States. *American Journal of Hygiene,* 1957, 65, 271–315.

Corcoran, A. C., Taylor, R. D., Page, I. H. Controlled observations on the effect of low sodium diet therapy in essential hypertension. *Circulation,* 1951, *3,* 1–16.

Court, J. M., Hill, G. J., Dunlop, M., & Boulton, T. J. C. Hypertension in childhood obesity. *Australian Paediactric Journal,* 1974, *10*:5, 296–300.

Cutilletta, A. F., Benjamin, M., Culpepper, W. S., & Oparil, S. Myocardial hypertrophy and ventricular performance in the absence of hypertension in the spontaneously hypertensive rat. *Journal of Molecular and Cellular Cardiology,* 1978, *10*:8, 689–693.

Cutilletta, A. F., Erinoff, L., Heller, A., Low, J., & Oparil, S. Development of left ventricular hypertrophy in young spontaneously hypertensive rats after peripheral sympathectomy. *Circulation Research,* 1977, *40*:4, 428–434.

Dahl, L. K. Salt and hypertension. *American Journal of Clinical Nutrition,* 1972, 25, 231–249.

Dahl, L. K., & Love, R. A. Etiological role of sodium chloride intake in essential hypertension in humans. *Journal of the American Medical Association,* 1957, *164,* 397–400.

Davignin, A., Rey, C., Payot, M., Biron, P., & Mongeau, J. G. Hemodynamic studies of labile essential hypertension. In M. I. New & C. S. Levine (eds.), *Juvenile hypertension.* New York: Raven Press, 1977.

Day, M. D., & Roach, A. G. Central alpha and beta adrenoreceptors modifying arterial blood pressure and heart rate in conscious cats. *British Journal of Pharmacology,* 1974, *51*:3, 325–333.

DeBacker, G. M., Kornitzer, F., Kittel, M., et al. Relation between coronary-prone behavior pattern, excretion of urinary catecholamines, heart rate, and heart rhythm. *Preventive Medicine*, 1979, 8:1, 14–22.

deCastro, F. J., Biesbroeck, R., Erickson, C., Farrell, P., Leong, W., Murphy, D., & Green, R. Hypertension in adolescents. *Clinical Pediatrics*, 1976, 15:1, 24–26.

Dembroski, T. M., & MacDougall, J. M. Stress effect of affiliation preferences among subjects possessing the Type A coronary prone behavior pattern. *Journal of Personality and Social Psychology*, 1978, 36:1, 23–33.

Dole, V. P., Dahl, L. K., Cotzias, G. C., Eder, H. A., & Krebs, M. E. Dietary treatment of hypertension: Clinical and metabolic studies of patients on the rice–fruit diet. *Journal of Clinical Investigation*, 1950, 29, 1189–1206.

Dube, S. K., Kapoor, S., Ratner, H., & Tunick, F. L. Blood pressure studies in black children. *American Journal of Diseases in Children*, 1975, 129:10, 1177–1180.

Emurian, H. H., Emurian, C. S., & Brady, J. V. Effects of pairing contingency on behavior in a three person programmed environment. *Journal of the Experimental Analysis of Behavior*, 1978, 29, 319–329.

Engel, B. T., & Bickford, A. F. Response specificity: stimulus-response and individual-response specificity in essential hypertensives. *Archives of General Psychiatry*, 1961, 5, 478–489.

Falkner, B., Onesti, G., Angelakos, E. T., Fernandes, M., & Langman, C. Cardiovascular response to mental stress in normal adolescents with hypertensive parents. *Hypertension*, 1979, 1:1, 23–30.

Farquhar, J. W., Maccoby, N., Wood, P. D., Alexander, J. K., Breitrose, H., Brown, B. W., Hashell, W. L., McAlister, A. L., Meyer, A. T., Nash, J. D., & Stein, M. P.Community education for cardiovascular health. *Lancet*, 1977, 1:8023, 1192–1195.

Feinleib, M., Garrison, R., Borhani, N. O., Rosenman, R., & Christian, J. Studies of hypertension in twins. In O. Paul (ed.), *Epidemiology and control of hypertension*. New York: Grune & Stratton, 1975.

Finnerty, F. A., Shaw, L. W., & Himmelsback, C. Hypertension in the inner city: II. Detection and follow-up. *Circulation*, 1973, 47, 76–78.

Frank, G. C., Farris, R. P., Mayor, C. R., Webber, L. S., & Berenson, G. S. Infant feeding patterns and their relationship to cardiovascular risk factor variables in the first year of life. Unpublished manuscript, The Bogalusa Heart Study, 1981.

Friedman, M., Rosenman, R. H ., Straus, R., et al. The relationship of behavior pattern A to the state of the vasculature: A study of 51 autopsied subjects. *American Journal of Medicine*, 1968, 44, 525–537.

Frolich, E. D. Hemodynamics of hypertension. In J. Genest, E. Koin, & O. Kuchel (eds.), *Hypertension: Physiology and treatment*. New York: McGraw-Hill, 1977.

Guzicki, J., & Coates, T. J. Cue-controlled relaxation for the classroom teacher. *Journal of School Psychology*, 1979, 18, 17–24.

Harlan, W. R., Oberman, A., Mitchel, R. E., & Graybiel, A. A 30-year study of blood pressure in a white male cohort. In G. Onesti, K. E. Kim, & J. H.

Mayer (eds.), *Hypertension: Mechanisms and management*. New York: Grune & Stratton, 1973.

Harlan, W. R., Osborne, R. K., & Graybiel, A. Prognostic value of the cold pressor test and the basal blood pressure. *American Journal of Cardiology*, 1964, *13*, 683–687.

Haynes, S. G., Feinleib, M., & Kannel, W. B. The relationship of psychosocial factors to coronary heart disease in the Framingham study. III. Eight year incidence of coronary heart disease. *American Journal of Epidemiology*, 1980, *111*:1, 37–58.

Haynes, S. G., Feinleib, M., Levine, S., Scotch, N., & Kannel, W. B. The relationship of the psychosocial factors to coronary heart disease. II. Prevalence of coronary heart disease. *American Journal of Epidemiology*, 1978, *104*, 384–402.

Haynes, S. G., Levine, S., Scotch, N., Feinleib, M., & Kannel, W. B. The relationship of psychosocial factors to coronary heart disease in Framingham study. I & II. *American Journal of Epidemiology*, 1978, *107*:5, 362–402.

Heyden, S., Bartel, A. G., Hanes, C. G., & McDonough, J. R. Elevated blood pressure levels in adolescents, Evans County, Georgia. *Journal of the American Medical Association*, 1969, *11*, 1683–1689.

Hines, E. A. Reaction of blood pressure of 400 school children to standard stimulus. *Journal of the American Medical Association*, 1937, *108*, 1249–1250.

Holland, W. W., & Beresford, S. A. A. Factors influencing blood pressure in children. In O. Paul (ed.), *Epidemiology and control of hypertension*. New York: Grune & Stratton, 1975, 375–383.

Horan, M. J., Kennedy, H. L., & Padgett, N. E. Do borderline hypertensive patients have labile blood pressure? *Annals of Internal Medicine*, 1981, *94*, 466–468.

Insel, P., & Chadwick, J. Conceptual barriers to the treatment of chronic disease. Using pediatric hypertension as an example. In T. J. Coates, A. C. Petersen, & C. Perry (eds.), *Adolescent health: Crossing the barriers*. New York: Academic Press, in press.

Jenkins, C. D., Zyzanski, S. J., & Rosenman, R. H. Risk of new myocardial infarction in middle-aged men with manifest coronary heart disease. *Circulation*, 1976, *53*:2, 342–347.

Kass, E. H., Zinner, S. H., Margolius, H. S., Yhu, L., Rosner, B., & Donner, A. Familial aggregation of blood pressure and urinary Kallikrein in early childhood. In O. Paul (ed.), *Epidemiology and control of hypertension*. New York: Grune & Stratton, 1975.

Kilcoyne, M. M., Richter, R. W., & Alsup, P. A. Adolescent hypertension: Detection and prevalence. *Circulation*, 1974, *50*:4, 758–764.

Klein, B. E., Hennikens, C. G., Jesse, M. J., Gourley, J. E., & Blumenthal, S. Longitudinal studies of blood pressure in offspring of hypertensive mothers. In O. Paul (ed.) *Epidemiology and control of hypertension*. New York: Grune & Stratton, 1975.

Kohlstaedt, K. G., Moser, M., Francis, T., Meel, J., & Moore, F. Panel discussion on genetic and environmental factors in human hypertension. *Circulation*, 1968, *17*, 728–742.

Kotchen, J. M., Dotchen, T. A., Schwertman, N. L., & Kuller, L. H. Blood pressure distributions of urban adolescents. *American Journal of Epidemiology*, 1974, *99*, 315–324.

Krantz, D. D., Schaeffer, M. A., Daria, J. E., Dembroski, T. M., & MacDougall, J. M. Investigation of the extent of coronary atherosclerosis, Type A behavior, and cardiovascular response to social interaction. *Psychophysiology*, in press.

Lacey, J. I., & Lacey, B. C. The law of initial value in the longitudinal study of autonomic constitution: Reproducibility of autonomic responses and response patterns over a four-year interval. *Annals of the New York Academy of Sciences*, 1962, *98*, 1257–1290.

Langford, H. G., & Watson, R. L. A study of the urinary sodium, salt taste threshold, and blood pressure resemblance of siblings. *Johns Hopkins Medical Journal*, 1972, *131*, 143–146.

Langford, H. G., & Watson, R. L. Electrolytes, environment, and blood pressure. *Clinical Science and Molecular Medicine*, 1973, *45*, 111s–113s.

Langford, H. G., & Watson, R. L. Electrolytes and hypertension. In O. Paul (ed.), *Epidemiology and control of hypertension*. New York: Grune & Stratton, 1975.

Langford, H. G., Watson, R. L., & Douglas, B. H. Factors affecting blood pressure in population groups. *Transactions of the Association of American Physicians*, 1968, *81*, 135–146.

Lauer, R. M., Filer, L. J., Reiter, M. A., & Clarke, W. R. Blood pressure, salt preference, salt threshold, and relative weight. *American Journal of Diseases in Children*, 1976, *130*:5, 493–497.

Lauer, R. M., Bartner, R. Coronary risk factors in children. In J. G. A. T. Hautvast & H. A. Valkenburg (eds.), *Atherosclerosis and the child*. Rotterdam: Erasmus University Press, 1977.

Littler, W. A., Honour, A. J., & Sleight, P. Direct arterial pressure, pulse rate, and electrocardiogram during micturition and defecation in unrestricted man. *American Heart Journal*, 1974, *88*, 205–210.

Littler, W. A., West, M. J., Honour, A. J., & Sleight, P. The variability of arterial pressure. *American Heart Journal*, 1978, *95*:2, 180–186.

Londe, S., Bourgoigne, J. J., Robson, A. M., & Goldring, D. Hypertension in apparently normal children. *Journal of Pediatrics*, 1971, *78*, 569–577.

Malmo, R. B., & Shagass, C. Physiologic study of symptom mechanisms in psychiatric patients under stress. *Psychosomatic Medicine*, 1949, *11*, 25–29.

Manuck, S. B., Corse, C. C., & Winkelman, P. A. Behavioral correlates of individual differences in blood pressure reactivity. *Journal of Psychosomatic Research*, 1979, *23*:4, 281–288.

Matthews, K. A., Glass, D. C., Rosenman, R. H., & Bortner, R. W. Competitive drive, pattern A, and coronary heart disease: A further analysis of some data from the Western Collaborative Group Study. *Journal of Chronic Diseases*, 1977, *30*:8, 489–498.

Miall, W. E., & Lovell, H. G. Relation between change in blood pressure and age. *British Medical Journal*, 1967, *2*, 660–664.

Miller, R. A., & Shekelle, R. B. Blood pressure in tenth grade students. *Circulation*, 1976, *54*:6, 993–1000.

Mueller, T. E., & Brown, G. E. Hourly rhythms in blood pressure in persons' with normal and elevated pressures. *Annals of Internal Medicine*, 1930, *3*, 1190–1195.

National Center for Health Statistics. *Hypertension and hypertensive vascular disease in adults, United States, 1960–1962*. Washington, D.C.: U.S. Government Printing Office, 1966, Vital and health statistics series 11, No. 13.

National Center for Health Statistics. *Blood pressure levels of children 6–11 years*. Washington, D.C.: U.S. Government Printing Office, 1973, publication (HRA) 74-1617, Vital and health statistics series 11, No. 135.

National Center for Health Statistics. *Blood pressures of youths 12–17 years*. Washington, D.C.: U.S. Government Printing Office, 1977, publication (HRA) 77-1645, Vital and health statistics series 11, No. 163.

Paffenbarger, R. S., Thorne, M. C., & Wing, A. L. Chronic diseases in former college students. VIII. Characteristics of youths predisposing to hypertension in later years. *American Journal of Epidemiology*, 1968, *88*, 25–32.

Paul, O. *Epidemiology and control of hypertension*. New York: Grune & Stratton, 1975.

Perloff, D., & Sokolow, M. The representative blood pressure: Usefulness of office, basal, home, and ambulatory readings. *Cardiovascular Medicine*, 1978, *3*, 655–668.

Pickering, O. W. *The nature of essential hypertension*. New York: Grune & Stratton, 1961.

Pooling Project Research Group. *The relationship of blood pressure, serum cholesterol, smoking habit, relative weight, and ECG abnormalities to incidence of major coronary events*. Dallas, Tex.: American Heart Association Monograph, 1978.

Reisin, E., Abel, R., Modau, M., Silverberg, D. S., Eliahon, H. E., & Modan, B. Effect of weight loss without salt restriction on the reduction of blood pressure in overweight hypertensive patients. *New England Journal of Medicine*, 1978, *298*:1, 1–6.

Rosenman, R. H., Brand, R. J., Sholtz, R. I., & Friedman, M. Multivariate prediction of coronary heart disease during 8.5 follow-up in the Western Collaborative Group Study. *American Journal of Cardiology*, 1976, *37*, 902–910.

Sannerstedt, R., Bjure, J., & Varnaushas, E. Correlation between echocardiographic changes and systemic hemodynamics in human arterial hypertension. *American Journal of Cardiology*, 1970, *26*, 117–122.

Schwartz, H., & Leitch, C. J. Differences in mean adolescent blood pressure by age, sex, ethnic origin and familial tendency. *Journal of School Health*, 1975, *45*, 76–82.

Siegel, J. M., & Leitch, C. J. Assessment of the Type A behavior pattern in adolescents. *Psychosomatic Medicine*, 1981, *43*, 45–56.

Sinaiko, A. R., & Mirkin, B. L. Clinical pharmacology of anti-hypertensive drugs in children. *Pediatric Clinics of North America*, 1978, *25*:1, 137–157.

Sokolow, M., Werdegar, D., Kain, H. K., & Hinman, A. T. Relationship between level of blood pressure measured casually and by portable recorder and severity of complications in essential hypertension. *Circulation*, 1966, *34*, 279–298.

Sokolow, M., Werdegar, D., Perloff, D. B., Cowan, R. M., & Brenenstuhl, H. Preliminary studies relating portably recorded blood pressures to daily life events in patients with essential hypertension. In M. Koster, H. Musaph, & P. Visser (eds.), *Psychosomatics in essential hypertension*. New York: Karger, 1970.

Spiga, R., & Petersen, A. C. The coronary-prone behavior pattern in early adolescence. Paper presented at the meetings of the American Educational Research Association, Boston, 1981.

Stamler, J., Stamler, R., Riadlinger, W. S., Algera, G., & Roberts, R. H. Hypertension screening of one million Americans. *Journal of the American Medical Association*, 1976, *235:*21, 2299–2306.

Stine, O. C., Hepner, R., & Greenstreet, R. Correlation of blood pressure with skinfold thickness and protein levels. *American Journal of Diseases of Children*, 1975, *129:*8, 905–911.

Surgeon General of the United States. *Healthy people: The Surgeon General's report on health promotion and disease prevention*. Washington, D.C.: Public Health Service, 1979 DHEW (PHS) Publication No. 79-55071.

Task Force on Blood Pressure Control. Report. *Pediatrics*, 1977, *59*, 797–820, supplement.

Tuthill, R. W., & Calabrese, E. J. Elevated sodium levels in public drinking water as a contributor to elevated blood pressure levels in the community. *Archives of Environmental Health*, 1979, *34:*4, 197–203.

Tuthill, R. W., & Calabrese, E. J. Drinking water sodium and blood pressure in children: A second look. *American Journal of Public Health*, 1981, *71*, 722–729.

Tyroler, H. A., Heyden, S., et al. Weight and hypertension: Evans County studies of blacks and whites. In O. Paul (ed.), *Epidemiology and control of hypertension*. New York: Grune & Stratton, 1975.

Voors, A. W., Foster, T. A., Frericks, R. R., Webber, L. S., & Berenson, B. I. Studies of blood pressures in children, ages 5–14 years, in a total biracial community: The Bogalusa Heart Study. *Circulation*, 1976, *54*, 319–327.

Voors, A. W., Sklor, M. C., Hunter, S. MacD., & Berenson, G. S. Cardiovascular risk factors in children and coronary related behavior. In T. S. Coates, A. C. Petersen, & C. Perry (eds.), *Promoting adolescent health: A dialogue in research and practice*. New York: Academic Press, 1982.

Waldron, I., Hickey, A., McPherson, C., Butensky, A., Gruss, L., Overall, K., Schmade, A., & Wohlmuth, D. Type A behavior pattern: Relationship to variation in blood pressure, parental characteristics, and academic and social activities of students. *Journal of Human Stress*, 1980, *6:*1, 16–27.

Willett, W. C. Drinking water sodium and blood pressure: A cautious view of the "second look." *American Journal of Public Health*, 1981, *71*, 729–732.

Zahka, K. G., Neill, C. A., Kidd, L., Cutilletta, M. A., & Cutilletta, A. F. Cardiac involvement in adolescent hypertension: Echocardiographic determination of myocardial hypertrophy. *Hypertension*, in press.

Zinner, S. H., Levy, P. S., & Kass, E. H. Familial aggregation of blood pressure in childhood. *New England Journal of Medicine*, 1971, *284*, 401–404.

CHAPTER **5**

Biobehavioral Effects of Pediatric Hospitalization

Belinda Traughber, Ph.D.
Michael F. Cataldo, Ph.D.

Introduction

Behavioral pediatrics integrates behavioral science principles and technology with pediatric medicine. As such, behavioral pediatrics can be conceptualized into three distinct categories: (1) the treatment of children's behavior problems through a pediatric clinical setting (e.g., an ambulatory pediatric outpatient service); (2) the use of behavioral procedures to remediate a diagnosed medical problem, usually by direct modification of the pathology (e.g., training external sphincter control in spina bifida pediatric patients so that they may achieve continence); and (3) reducing the iatrogenic behavioral and biological effects of quality medical care. The first two categories are addressed elsewhere in this book. This chapter will deal with the third category by focusing on the hospitalized child.

For children, the hospital environment contains a bewildering array of unfamiliar people, procedures, and machinery and is a place in which they encounter a variety of aversive events. Many children have been noted to exhibit maladaptive reactions to the experience of hospitalization either during their hospital stay or once they have returned home. Although admission automatically implies some physical dysfunction with its concomitant pain and/or distress, at least some portion of children's reactions can be attributed to the aversive properties of the setting itself (see Chapman, Loeb, & Gibbons, 1956; Ferguson, 1979; Gellert, 1958; Haller,

Support for the preparation of this paper was provided in part by Grant 917 from Maternal and Child Health. This work is a joint effort of the Kennedy Institute and the Behavioral Medicine Program of The Johns Hopkins School of Medicine.

Talbert, & Dombro, 1967; Prugh, Staub, Sands, Kirschbaum, & Lenihan, 1953; Vernon, Foley, Sipowicz, & Schulman, 1965; Visintainer & Wolfer, 1975; Wolfer & Visintainer, 1979). The potential magnitude of this problem is not trivial. A 1979 survey by the American Hospital Association of 6321 hospitals indicated that pediatric services provided over 55,000 beds. Based on an 80 percent census, this translates into over 16 million pediatric patient bed days per year.

In order to consider properly a behavioral pediatrics approach to the iatrogenic effects of hospitalization, those behavioral principles relevant to the problem should be detailed at the onset. Our premise is that the hospital environment provides a variety of aversive events, especially to the pediatric patient. Accordingly, the behavioral research literatures on aversive stimulation will be reviewed briefly. Next, research on the hospitalized child will be discussed both in light of theories of development and how such previous research relates to principles of behavior. Unfortunately, most of the research on the problems encountered by hospitalized children has not been based on well-documented basic behavioral research on aversive stimulation. The preliminary research that has been so based will be presented in detail, along with considerations for future investigations as a final section to the chapter.

Previous Research on Aversive Stimulation

Controllability and Predictability of Aversive Stimuli

Aversive stimulation has been demonstrated to produce a variety of behavioral and biological reactions in humans and animals (Badia, Culbertson, & Harsh, 1973; Miller & Seligman, 1973; Reim, Glass, & Singer, 1971; Seligman, 1975). Behavioral reactions are typified initially by escape or avoidance responses. When these are unsuccessful, a generalized suppression of behavior occurs. This suppression of behavior is speculated to be a function of the organism learning that its responses and the aversive event are independent (e.g., learned helplessness; Seligman, 1975). Two factors that have been demonstrated to affect behavioral reactions to aversive stimuli are the relative controllability and/or predictability of the stimuli.

Aversive stimuli that are used commonly in laboratory experiments are shock and noise. Generally, animals and humans show a preference for signaled versus unsignaled and contingent versus noncontingent aversive stimuli. Badia, et al., (1973) examined the relative aversiveness of signaled and unsignaled shock for rats and found that they chose signaled shock that was four to nine times longer in duration or two to three times more intense than unsignaled shock. Throughout their study, the unsignaled shock was left unchanged in intensity and duration and a time-out component was included each hour to ensure that subjects experienced the unsignaled condition. Their study provided evidence for the theory of the "safety signal hypothesis" (Seligman, 1975) in which stimuli that identify periods of time free from aversive stimulation acquire reinforcing properties. In a later study (Badia & Culbertson, 1972), the relative aversiveness of signaled versus unsignaled escapable and inescapable shock was examined. Results showed that rats preferred signaled shock in both conditions. It has been demonstrated widely that stimulus identification of shock-free periods suppresses avoidance responding (Rescorla & LoLordo, 1965), that the duration of the shock-free period is related to its suppressive effect on avoidance (Weissman & Litner, 1971), and that operant responses can be maintained by stimuli that identify shock-free periods (Sidman, 1962).

Learning and task performance have been shown to be impaired subsequent to the presentation of aversive stimuli (Miller & Seligman, 1973; Reim et al., 1971). This is of particular concern when considering the impact of hospitalization on children.

Biological Reactions to Aversive Stimuli

These can be observed in cardiovascular, endocrine, and gastrointestinal changes. Although the direction of these reactions is similar across persons, the amount of change varies. Such measurements, therefore, are most useful in single-subject designs until normative data become more available. A review of the field of psychosocial stimuli and adrenal cortical response (Rubin & Mandell, 1966) shows that increased levels of thyroid and related substances result on exposure to trauma, noise, sensory deprivation, and other aversive stimuli in both animals and humans.

The predictable stimulation of the adrenal cortical system provides one of the most promising means of assessing the impact of aversive events on humans. Among other functions, the central nervous system is involved in the regulation of secretion of pituitary adrenocorticotropic hormone (ACTH). The pituitary–adrenal system is stimulated under conditions in which the organism is threatened, thus causing increased ACTH release and subsequent increased secretion of adrenocortical hormones. This can be measured in the urinary excretion or plasma levels of 17-hydroxycorticosteroids (17-OHCS) (Kagan & Levi, 1975). Given the routine collection of urine and plasma samples in hospitals, this measure is convenient and has been used in a variety of studies examining the reactions of adults to hospitalization.

Price, Thaler, & Mason (1957) examined the relationship of preoperative emotional states and adrenal cortical activity in adult cardiac and pulmonary surgery patients, comparing excretion levels of 17-OHCS to psychologists' and psychiatrists' ratings of anxiety and degree of discomfort involvement. The adrenocortical hormone levels were measured through diurnal blood samples drawn in a period ranging from 21 days before surgery to the morning of surgery, with all subjects having blood samples drawn on the day prior to surgery. Normal subjects in the laboratory had an average of 12 mg/100 ml plasma of 17-OHCS. In contrast, the average of the 63 surgical patients at 8 A.M. of the day before surgery was 17.7 mg/100 ml plasma. On patients rated as highly anxious by both psychiatrists and psychologists, the mean levels were 21 and 23 mg/100 ml. Although in acute stress situations peak plasma 17-OHCS ranging to 70 mg/100 ml or above may be seen, levels in the range of 20 to 30 mg/100 ml represent significant increases in adrenocortical activity in longer-term stressful circumstances.

In another study, Mason, Sachar, Fishman, Hamburg, & Handlon (1965) measured 17-OHCS levels in 60 normal adult volunteers during admission to a hospital-controlled research ward. Their levels were significantly higher the day of admission than later in hospitalization, which suggests that these changes were part of the subjects' psychoendocrine response to environmental change. There was a considerable range of group and individual differences, but all subjects maintained their relative positions with respect to 17-OHCS levels. The mean change from day one to the second week of the study was 7.2 to 6 mg per day (a drop of about 17 percent), which was attributed to the effect of a novel and unpredictable environment.

Fishman, Hamburg, Handlon, Mason, & Sachar (1962) demonstrated increases in 17-OHCS levels for a moderate-stress group, as compared to a control group. Persky, Korchin, Basowitz, Board, Sabshin, Hamburg, & Grinker (1959) also demonstrated that the urinary excretion of 17-OHCS of anxious patients was higher than normals and their plasma level lower. Increased urinary catecholamine excretion also has been demonstrated for medical examination (Bliss, Migeon, Branch, & Samuels, 1956; Ulvedal, Smith, & Welch, 1963), hospital admission (Nelson, Masuda, & Holmes, 1966), and anticipation of thoracic surgery (Price et al., 1957).

Other measures available to assess biological effects of aversive stimulation in humans are the Palmar Sweat Index (Melamed & Siegel, 1975), which is a plastic-impression method that permits quantification of active hand sweat-gland activity. The sweat glands of the hand are believed to be affected primarily by emotional factors and not such other variables as temperature. Thus, this measure provides data on transitory physiological arousal. The electrical conductivity of the skin as measured by galvanic skin resistance (GSR) is another indicator of sweat secretion that frequently is used. Other typical reactions include accelerated pulse rate, increased blood pressure, dryness of the throat and mouth, insomnia, frequent urination, diarrhea, indigestion, queasiness of the stomach, vomiting, migraine headaches, and increased muscle tension as measured by electromyography (EMG).

With regard to the cardiovascular system, anticipating a shock-avoidance schedule has been shown to result in elevated blood pressure with a decrease or no change in heart rate (Anderson & Brady, 1971; Anderson & Tosheff, 1973). Both rhesus (Forsyth, 1969) and squirrel monkeys (Herd, Morse, Kelleher, & Jones, 1969) have developed hypertensive blood pressure levels under conditions of responding to avoid aversive stimulation. In other studies, gastric stomach lesions have occurred as a result of animals receiving unavoidable shocks (Moot, Cebulla, & Crabtree, 1970; Weiss, 1971). Unavoidable aversive stimulation also has been shown to result in decreased levels of norepinephrine in the brain (Weiss, Stone, & Harrell, 1970; Weiss, Glazer, & Pohorecky, 1976) and subsequent decrements in the ability to learn (Glazer, Weiss, Pohorecky, & Miller, 1975; Weiss, Glazer, Pohorecky, Brick, & Miller, 1975).

Mitigation of Aversive Stimuli

Thus, research has shown that aversive stimulation can result in biological reactions, suppression of various types of behavior, and retarded learning. Conditions that have been shown to mitigate these effects for uncontrollable aversive stimuli are the presentation of competing positive events (Pavlov, 1927; Brady, 1955) or making the occurrence of the aversive stimulus more predictable. A more detailed discussion of this issue is presented in a review by Cataldo, Jacobs, & Rogers (in press).

With regard to conditions that mitigate aversive events, however, considerable further study is needed to clarify the reactions to aversive stimulation of various types. For example, a study by Friedman, Ader, & Glasgow (1965) on susceptibility to disease compared the effects of signaled and unsignaled shock. Four groups of mice were inoculated with virus and four with placebo. Prior to inoculation each mouse was placed in one of four treatment conditions: paired signal and aversive event; unsignaled aversive event; signal only; placement in experimental chamber only. Four days later, susceptibility to virus was assessed as indexed by weight loss. The virus-inoculated group that had received a signaled noxious event was the only one to show significant weight loss. This is a strong argument for the simultaneous measurement of biological and behavioral reactions to aversive stimuli to assess their relative impact. The relationship between somatic and behavioral effects of stress must be examined further.

Research on Hospitalized Children

Stress

Unfortunately, while much of the recently reported procedures in behavioral pediatrics have been based on basic behavior research similar to the type just discussed, this has not been the approach taken with research on iatrogenic effects. Much of the literature on children and hospitalization typifies their actions within the setting as responses to the "stress of hospitalization." Unfortunately, the concept is a broad one, and many writers fail to formulate operational definitions of the particular stressors under consideration. Lazarus, in *The International Encyclopedia of the Social Sciences* (1968), writes; "Stress suggests excessive demands that produce disturbances of physiological, social and psychological systems. . . . The term is thus loose in that it is applied to a host of phenomena related only by their common analogy with the engineering concept" (p. 338).

An approach to the definition of stress that is favored for medical and psychological research uses the model of biological–social homeostasis. This suggests that all living organisms work to maintain a state of homeostasis or equilibrium. Excessive or insufficient input of stimuli threaten equilibrium and function as stressors. The measurement of stress in humans is complicated by the individual variability in the range of what constitutes "reasonable" levels of stimuli. For further discussion of the concept of biological–social homeostasis, see Margetts (1954) and Toch & Hastorf (1955).

A more popular definition of stress is Selye's: "Stress is the state manifested by a specific syndrome which consists of all the nonspecifically induced changes within a biologic system" (Selye, 1976).

Aversive Stimulation

Because stress can signify positive as well as aversive events, the experiences of hospitalized children will be examined in terms of aversive stimulation rather than the more general concept of stress. A variety of events associated with hospitalization are noted to be aversive to children. Among those cited in the literature are separation from home and parents; surgical procedures; medical procedures of a traumatic, painful nature; immobilization required in the case of some illnesses; danger of death; and unfamiliarity of the hospital setting (Nagera, 1978). Gellert (1958) described children's reactions to hospitalization as follows:

> The stress of hospitalization for children is manifested in a number of ways. Children cry, whine, or scream; they cling tenaciously to their parents; they eat or sleep poorly; they struggle against treatment and resist taking medications; they are tense and fearful; they become silent, sad and withdrawn. They may show an increase in regressive or compulsive behavior; they may become destructive of their environment, or even themselves. [p. 125]

This description fits the focus of concern in the present, as does Chapman et al.'s description (1956) of posthospital upset:

> There is a wide variety of symptom and personality problems which may follow traumatic hospital experiences. Among the more common reactions are (a) eating problems with either refusal or overeating; (b) sleep disturbances, such as insomnia, nightmares or phobias of the dark; (c) enuresis, or fecal soiling; (d) regression to earlier levels of behavior and the loss of previously achieved levels of training and social functioning; (e) tics; (f) depression, restlessness and anxiety; (g) terror of hospitals, medical personnel, hypodermic needles, etc.; (h) death fears; (i) mute autistic regression to uncommunicative states, or frightened withdrawal from contact with people; (j) hypochondriacal body over-concern, or actual delusions about body functions; (k) hysterical symptoms, such as aphonia after tonsillectomy. [p. 84]

Estimates of the incidence of these problems remain highly variable, with several early studies reporting manifestation of problem behaviors in 10 percent to 35 percent of hospitalized children (Jessner, Blom, & Waldfogel, 1952; Prugh et al., 1953). More recently, Cassell (1965) reported at least slight psychological upset in as many as 92 percent of the children studied. Although adverse reactions can be expected to result from pain associated with the illness or trauma for which a child is admitted, there is evidence that the hospital experience itself produces anxiety for the child, irrespective of the reason for the hospitalization (Skipper & Leonard, 1968).

Much of the available literature addressing the impact of hospitalization on children is of an anecdotal nature; however, increasing emphasis is being placed on empirical assessment to determine the extent and nature of the problems and their controlling variables. In a comprehensive review of the earlier literature, Vernon et al. (1965) focused their attention on the following "determinants of psychological upset": unfamiliarity of the hospital setting; separation; interpersonal relationships during hospitalization, sensory–motor restrictions; children's conceptions of hospitalization; age;

parent–child relationships and prehospital personality; emotional responses of parents; previous hospitalization; previous separation; sex; characteristics of the disability and treatment; and miscellaneous hospital arrangements and procedures. They determined that only four of the factors were investigated with sufficient thoroughness to warrant a summary of the data. These were unfamiliarity with the hospital setting, separation, age, and prehospital personality. The results of a number of studies indicated that preparing the child for surgery or hospitalization by providing information about procedures tends to decrease the incidence of psychological upset in the posthospital period, but the relationship between psychological preparation and responses during hospitalization was not clear. Data on separation from parents/home indicated that it contributed to upset both during and immediately following hospitalization but was unlikely to have long-term consequences for emotional adjustment. Parent–child contacts during the separation appeared to mitigate the effects. There was a curvilinear relationship between age of the child and psychological upset. Children between approximately six months and three to four years of age appeared to be particularly vulnerable to upset during hospitalization, with younger infants and older children appearing less vulnerable. Some evidence was presented that poor prior adjustment is likely to be associated with more frequent or more severe upset both during and following hospitalization.

Separation Anxiety

Separation from their parents is frequently noted as a source of psychological upset for hospitalized children and is cited often as the major source of stress for children under the age of five (Bowlby, 1973; Nagera, 1978). There is little research available that attempts to differentiate the impact of separation from parents from other sources of stress on hospitalized children. Nor is there research that attempts to determine whether separation anxiety is anything more than a hypothetical construct for the same findings from basic animal and human behavioral research just discussed. However, Bowlby (1973) provides extensive documentation of the effects of separation on nonhospitalized children. Many healthy children placed in nurseries, institutions, or brief foster care exhibit a wide range of distressed behaviors upon separation from the mother. The distressed behaviors typically follow three stages: protest, despair, and detachment. Behaviors that have been attributed to separation anxiety include sleep disturbances, increase in demands, tachycardia, palpitations, hyperventilation, diarrhea, vomiting, aphonia, disturbance of vision, enuresis, and encopresis. Severity of the stress appears to be affected by the age of the child, length of the separation and the child's prior experiences of separation. Children under the age of two and a half to three years suffer most severely from separation anxiety. Between the ages of three and five years, the child's capacity to tolerate separation increases. After the age of five years, very few children are affected adversely by brief separations. Nagera (1978) suggests that if the child is ill, in pain, frightened, or hurt he loses the capacity to tolerate separation and his behavior is regressive. Extended separation from the mother during the first year of life can result in marasmus. Prolonged separation for children up to the age of 18 months may result in delayed biological development, with concomitant irreversible damage to cognitive and intellectual functioning. The loss of stimulation provided by the mother is thought to be a major cause of such delays.

Conditions that appear to mitigate the separation anxiety are the presence of a familiar companion or, to a lesser extent, familiar possessions and mothering care from substitute mothers. These findings suggest that, prior to hospitalization, one should assess whether or not the child has acquired the capacity to separate from the mother and accept a mother substitute; if not, one should allow the mother to accompany the child during the hospitalization. The belief that mother substitutes can be helpful in alleviating in-hospital distress can be seen in staffing patterns in many hospitals, where one nurse is assigned to a child throughout the stay.

Schaffer (Schaffer, 1958; Schaffer & Callender, 1959) studied 25 healthy infants of various ages under the age of 12 months admitted to the hospital for elective surgery. The healthy children's responses to hospitalization were shown to be sharply differentiated by age. Children aged 28 weeks and younger showed no differentiation in their reactions to people, whereas those aged 28 to 51 weeks showed clinging to the mother and hostility toward strangers. All children exhibited sleep disturbances and night crying. As these children were not experiencing pain or illness when assessed, the authors concluded behavior disturbance to be due to separation anxiety.

If separation anxiety is accepted as a cause of some in-hospital distress, consideration should be given to the identification and moderation of this reaction. Recently, some hospitals have made arrangements for parents to sleep in with their children and participate in their care. Examination of such programs appears to be the most feasible means of isolating the impact of separation from parents on hospitalized children. There have been few attempts, however, to demonstrate experimentally the efficacy of this procedure in the alleviation of the stress of hospitalization for children, nor to determine whether the observed behaviors are described more correctly in the context of aversive stimulation occurring in a hospital, of which separation is only one component.

Fagin (1964) matched by age two groups of 30 children between the ages of 18 and 48 months and compared the effect of having the mother remain in the hospital with the children for a short hospitalization. For one group of children, the mother stayed overnight; for the other group, the mother visited daily. Children were compared on the basis of mothers' reports of their behavior at home. Mothers were interviewed prior to the hospitalization and at one week and one month after discharge. Their reports indicated that children whose mothers did not live in were markedly disturbed in comparison to their behavior prior to hospitalization. Specifically, the unaccompanied children were reported as being much more dependent and upset by brief separations than they were prior to hospitalization. Children whose mothers lived in with them showed none of these effects. Interviewers also rated the mothers' irritability, and it was noted that unaccompanied children with irritable mothers were affected even more by the separation. However, the groups of children were not matched for ailment or length of stay. Twenty-one of the accompanied children were in the hospital for a hernia operation or tonsillectomy and were out again within two days. Only nine of the unaccompanied children had a similar experience. Thirteen of these had respiratory or alimentary infections and stayed in the hospital for three to five days. Thus, though this study suggests that allowing the mother to accompany children in the hospital alleviates the adverse impacts of the experience, results may have been due to the varied length of stay or the child's physical condition. In addition, all outcome measures were based on the mother's report. The possibility that accompanying the child could affect the mother's objectivity in rating behavior also should be assessed.

Based on Bowlby's work (1969; 1973), the most important separation variables to be addressed first are age, sex, length of separation, and prior experiences of separation from parents. Perhaps the simplest way to approach the problem would be to study groups of children scheduled for elective surgery of matched types. This strategy, similar to the Fagin study (1964), is used extensively in studies of the effects of preparation for hospitalization and allows a measure of prior control over subject characteristics. Prescheduled hospital stays allow time to question the parents on the child's prior experiences of separation.

Conditions could be varied, such as allowing the parent to live in with the child and participate in the child's care, versus restricting the parents to usual hospital visiting hours. Among the children whose parents do not stay in the hospital, the effect of provision of substitute mothering care could be assessed by varying the staffing patterns to assign the same person to care for the child throughout the stay, compared to rotating primary caregivers. Ideally, one group would have the nurse or aide care for the

"largely wasted effort for professional staff." Preoperative techniques in use were (1) narrative explanation of hospital experience (61%); (2) printed material such as coloring books or story books (55%); (3) play therapy (48%); (4) filmed model depicting child's hospital experience (37%); (5) puppet show (21%); (6) specific behavioral techniques such as relaxation training and deep-breathing (16%); and (7) preadmission tours, a slide presentation, or meeting some of the staff prior to admission (27%). The greatest limitation appeared to be the percentage of children in the hospitals who typically received the available prehospital preparation. Reports ranged from zero to 100 percent, with an average of 42 percent. Thirty-four percent of the hospitals reported that prehospitalization preparation was provided to more than half the children admitted, and 48 percent reported providing preparation to less than half of pediatric admissions. This survey covered only pediatric hospitals and did not include general hospitals with pediatric wards, in which the use of special techniques for preparing children would reasonably be expected to be less infrequent.

The studies on preparing children for the experience of hospitalization appear to support research on the preference of organisms for signaled versus unsignaled aversive events; however, at least one disturbing study with adult patients must be noted. Suzanne Miller (1980) has described a theory of coping with aversive events that is termed the "blunting hypothesis" and is an extension of Seligman's safety signal hypothesis (1975). People are divided into two basic categories, blunters and monitors, based on their strategy of coping with danger. Blunters, when faced with a physical danger signal, remove themselves psychologically from the danger by "blunting" the psychological impact of physically present danger signals through cognitive strategies such as distraction, self-relaxation, or, more negatively, denial and detachment. Monitors, on the other hand, seek out information about the possible danger. Using a scale developed to differentiate the two groups, a group of gynecologic patients about to undergo colposcopy (a diagnostic procedure to check for presence of cancerous cells in the uterus) was divided into blunters and monitors. Half of each group then was given minimal information about the procedure and the other half given extensive detail. Self-report and physiological measures (pulse rate) of arousal were taken before, during, and after the procedure. In addition, the physician rated the women's anxiety through assessment of muscular tension during the examination. Patients then rated their subsequent discomfort for the five days following the procedure. Results indicated that the patients' level of arousal was reduced when the level of preparation was consistent with their coping style. However, the high-information groups showed increased subjective arousal across groups both before, immediately after, and in the five days following the procedure; however, the total distress produced by high information seemed to outweigh the distress produced by low information.

These results strongly suggest that further study is needed before endorsing the use of high-information preparation techniques for all patients.

Dealing with Painful Procedures

Most interventions designed to reduce the impact of hospitalization on children have dealt with patients suffering relatively minor illnesses (e.g., tonsillectomies). Their reactions may be substantially different from those of children undergoing more painful procedures. Katz, Kellerman, & Siegel (1980) developed an observational behavior rating scale to measure anxiety responses to painful bone-marrow aspirations in 115 children with cancer. The scale was designed to differentiate between high-anxiety and low-anxiety children as compared to nurse ratings. They found a significant relationship between age and both quantity and type of anxious behavior, with younger children tending to emit a greater variety of anxious behaviors over a longer period of time than older children. A developmental trend toward behavioral withdrawal and increased muscle tension with advancing age also was found. Girls tended to display higher levels of anxiety than did boys across age groups and to express this with comfort-seeking, as opposed to uncooperative, behavior. Age-by-sex interactions were absent. This study was particularly interesting because the children studied (cancer victims) represented a demographic cross-section of the population from which they were drawn and could be considered psychologically normal; thus, the impact of intense stress on generally adequately functioning children could be studied.

The investigation centered on the use of the Procedure Behavioral Rating Scale (PBRS), which originally consisted of 25 behavioral measures compiled by the authors. Items were eliminated that did not occur or occurred infrequently during 115 bone-marrow aspirations. One other item (groan) was eliminated because it failed to discriminate between age groups or "stress" groups (as identified by nurse ratings). The item of "questions" was eliminated because it correlated significantly but negatively with high-anxiety items, suggesting it was not indicative of anxiety but was anxiety mediating. Ratings were taken at four different periods: (1) when child was called from waiting room, until child reached door of treatment room; (2) when child entered treatment room, until child removed clothes; (3) when site was cleansed, anesthetic administered, and bone-marrow aspiration done, until needle was withdrawn; and (4) when bandage placed on site, until child left room. Though mean scores varied by age group, the fewest anxious behaviors occurred during period 1, increased in period 2, peaked in period 3, and then dropped in period 4 but remained at a level higher than period 1. Almost all (97%) of the children exhibited behavioral anxiety during the actual procedure, regardless of the number of procedures the child had undergone previously. The 13-item scale differentiated between high- and low-anxiety children, as measured by independent nurses' ratings, and identified quantitative and qualitative differences in anxiety as related to age and sex. Younger children exhibited consistently higher levels of distress than older children. Younger children ' also displayed a greater variety of anxious responses over a longer time span with less body control and more diffuse vocal protest. Girls were rated as more anxious than boys (similar to Melamed & Siegel, 1975). These sex differences were clear during the postprocedural phase but not during the actual procedure.

Behavioral Approaches to Intensive Care

Although a great deal of concern has been evidenced about the "intensive care syndrome" with adults (see Blachly & Starr, 1964; Egerton & Kay, 1964; Kornfeld, 1977; Kornfeld, Zimberg, & Malm, 1965; Lazarus & Hagens, 1968; McKegney, 1966), relatively little research has assessed the impact of the Intensive Care Unit (ICU) environment on children (Cataldo, Bessman, Parker, Pearson, & Rogers, 1979; Pearson, Cataldo, Tureman, Bessman, & Rogers, 1980; Shorkey & Taylor, 1973). As these children are at most risk for loss of life and can afford least to utilize their bodies' scarce resources to fight the impact of aversive environmental stimuli, more thorough examination of the impact of the hospital environment on their behavior is greatly needed.

Several studies indicate that, even for these highly traumatized children, relatively simple intervention techniques may alleviate the impact of the ICU. Although prehospital preparation is a technique unavailable to children admitted for acute illnesses or trauma, it frequently is possible to provide some measure of predictability after admission. Shorkey & Taylor (1973) presented anecdotal evidence that provision of discriminative stimuli for painful procedures decreased the anxiety responses of a 17-month-old girl suffering from severe burns. This child fought medical procedures, cried, and became extremely agitated when approached by staff members, refusing even to eat. This led them to conclude that staff members had become conditioned aversive stimuli through their association with the painful treatment. To aid the child in discriminating painful from social situations, nurses were instructed to wear red gowns and turn on red lights in the room for purely social conditions. For medical treatment, the nurses continued to wear their green gowns and were instructed not to interact

124 Pediatric and Adolescent Behavioral Medicine

with the child. No data were presented, but the authors reported that the child's anxiety responses under the social condition and during treatment procedures were decreased.

In a series of three studies on a pediatric intensive care unit (PICU), we have demonstrated that a simple environmental manipulation providing positive experiences (play activities) positively affected the behavior of the children (Cataldo et al., 1979; Pearson et al., 1980). Activity interventions resulted in increased attention, engagement, and positive affect and decreased inappropriate behavior. These studies are particularly encouraging because of their experimental and observational methodology.

In the first study (Cataldo et al., 1979), 99 patients ranging in age from two days to 22 years (mean, 6 years; median, 4 years) were observed over a two-month period. The length of stay for the observed patients ranged from one day to 11 months (mean, 4.9 days; median, 2 days). As neither the specific types of child behavior nor the environmental components that were interacting with that behavior could be predicted, specific target behaviors were not identified. Rather, in an assessment similar to the Resident Activity Manifest (Cataldo & Risley, 1974), observers recorded phrases describing the child's behavior across the categories of waking state; position; verbalizations from, to, and in the presence of the child; attention on eye contact; affective state; number and type of people within one meter of the bed; and activity. These behaviors were recorded in one-minute time samples. Across the two months of observation, slightly more than half of the children (54%) were in a sleeping/coma state but a large proportion were judged to be awake (11%) or awake and alert (35%). Of the children judged to be awake and alert, many more instances of negative (33%) than positive (3%) affective behaviors were demonstrated. More than half of the children displayed neutral affect (58%), and the most frequent category of what they were judged to be attending to was "nothing" (37%). For verbal behaviors, on 55 percent of the observations of awake and alert children someone (usually the nurse) spoke to the child; however, in 82 percent of the observations, no verbal behavior of the alert children was noted. Thus, though approximately one-third of the children on the PICU were in a state in which they could be assumed to be responsive to their environment, the majority of them were not doing or saying anything. Preliminary data analysis of a systematic replication currently in progress is showing the same general trends for child behavior during the day.

The second study (Cataldo et al., 1979) was designed to assess whether this behavior was the result of the children's physical condition and, if not, to assess the feasibility of increasing these children's interactions with their environment. A reversal design was employed to evaluate the effects of planned play-related activities on affect, attention, eye contact, interaction, and inappropriate behaviors. For some children, the activity intervention resulted in positive affective changes and reduced inappropriate behaviors, thus demonstrating that at least some portions of the behaviors of children in the PICU can be altered. These findings were replicated in a third study (Pearson et al., 1980) in which the duration of each condition was increased. For all 11 patients in the study, interaction was greater during the intervention than either before or after.

Another study has described extensively the environment of a neonatal ICU (Lawson, Daum, & Turkewitz, 1977). This investigation obtained an index of the density and distribution over 24-hour periods of the occurrence of sounds, the handling of infants, the level of illumination, and the sound-pressure levels in such a unit, with observations taken every 15 minutes. However, the experimenters did not note the behavior of the infants within that environment.

The observational system we have used on the PICU (Cataldo et al., 1979) appears to be a useful one for describing the hospital environment and children's actions within that environment. Future work should correlate this information with biological measures of the child's reactions to the environment. Since neither the child's physical status nor the medical procedures can be manipulated experimentally, research on interventions to lessen the impact of hospitalization on children will have to focus on specific aspects of the environment.

Summary and Future Considerations

If the assumption that hospital environments provide aversive stimulation to children is correct, then a considerable body of basic research exists about the behavioral and biological reactions to aversive conditions. This basic research can serve as the basis for selecting measures to assess whether hospital experiences produce behavioral and biological responses similar to those occurring when aversive stimulation is experimentally programmed. In addition, such basic research on conditions that mitigate the effects of aversive events can suggest intervention strategies for reducing the undesired outcomes of quality care on pediatric wards.

While a considerable amount of research has been reported on children's reactions to hospital environments, very few studies have reported data on child behavior, and fewer have employed measures of biological reactions. Clinical ratings, which comprise the majority of research-report data, are useful, but future research now can progress to more direct and sophisticated measures, especially in light of the basic research on aversive stimulation.

The use of biological reactions to hospital events not only will provide valuable insight into the aversive properties of the environment, but also will address directly the clinical importance of intervention strategies. Traditionally, rationales for psychosocial interventions have rested on suppositions about temporary loss of developmental skills, increases in disruptive and negative behaviors both during and after a hospital stay, and phobic-type reactions to future contacts with hospital environments and medical personnel. However, especially with the critically ill child, additional trauma caused by current hospital practices may place children at additional, significant clinical risk. That is, conditions of the hospital environment that present aversive stimulation or stimuli associated with aversive stimulation may increase risk factors in critical-care medicine.

Briefly, with regard to this point, response to trauma includes increased metabolic activity (Cuthbertson, 1930). This metabolic or neuroendocrine response to injury is believed to occur primarily for the restoration of homeostasis, particularly blood volume (Gann, 1976; Pirkle & Gann, 1976; Jarhult, 1973; Jarhult, Lundvall, Mellander, & Tibblin, 1972). However, this is not without cost to the patient, which includes increased oxygen consumption, energy needs, and protein breakdown (Baue, 1974). This hypermetabolic state, while necessary, does call upon finite oxygen and nutritional resources; resources which, for the critically ill patient, should not have to be used in response to environmental trauma as well. While the mechanisms are not understood completely, catecholamines have a direct relationship in mediating the hypermetabolic state (Harrison, Seaton, & Feller, 1967; Wilmore, Long, Mason, Skreen, & Pruitt, 1974). Therefore, elevations in catecholamine levels in response to environmental events may indicate an unwanted metabolic demand better reserved for response to physical trauma. Thus, consideration of how the hospital environment affects children should include the effects on their biological (and therefore medical) status as well as indices of psychological and behavioral changes.

Intervention strategies must never compromise the quality of medical care; however, the research to date on preparing children for hospitalization, making more predictable the occurrences of aversive events, and providing positive events on the hospital ward all have been conducted without disrupting routine or reducing medical care. Conversely, future research should not rest solely on clinical outcome. The process affecting behavioral and biological reactions needs to be understood better. This will permit the design of more effective intervention strategies and will advance basic knowledge.

Thus, the pediatric hospital may provide not only a setting to study methods for further improving the medical status of the patient and reducing psychological risk of hospitalization, but also a unique opportunity to study the effects of aversive events on children. Such basic research on children would not be approved by our current ethical standards if conducted in the laboratory; but, on the hospital ward, a natural and necessary laboratory setting exists for the better understanding of and improvement in child health and development.

References

American Hospital Association. *Hospital Statistics*. Chicago: American Hospital Association, 1979.

Anderson, D. E., & Brady, J. V. Pre-avoidance blood pressure elevations accompanied by heart rate decreases in the dog. *Science*, 1971, *172*, 595–597.

Anderson, D. E., & Tosheff, J. Cardiac output and total peripheral resistance changes during pre-avoidance periods in the dog. *Journal of Applied Psychology*, 1973, *34*, 650–654.

Badia, P., & Culbertson, S. The relative aversiveness of signaled versus unsignaled escapable and inescapable shock. *Journal of the Experimental Analysis of Behavior*, 1972, *17*, 463–471.

Badia, P., Culbertson, S., & Harsh, J. Choice of longer or stronger signaled shock over shorter or weaker unsignaled shock. *Journal of the Experimental Analysis of Behavior*, 1973, *19*, 25–32.

Baue, A. E. The energy crisis in surgical patients. *Archives of Surgery*, 1974, *109*, 249–250.

Blachly, P. H., & Starr, A. Post-cardiotomy delirium. *American Journal of Psychiatry*, 1964, *121*, 371–375.

Bliss, E. L., Migeon, C. J., Branch, C. H. H., & Samuels, L. T. Reaction of the adrenal cortex to emotional stress. *Psychosomatic Medicine*, 1956, *18*, 56–76.

Bowlby, J. *Attachment and loss. Vol. 1: Attachment*. New York, N.Y.: Basic Books, 1969.

Bowlby, J. *Attachment and loss. Vol. 2: Separation*. New York, N.Y.: Basic Books, 1973.

Brady, J. V. Extinction of a conditioned "fear" response as a function of reinforcement schedules for competing behavior. *Journal of Psychology*, 1955, *40*, 25–34.

Cassell, S. E. The effect of brief puppet therapy upon the emotional responses of children undergoing cardiac catheterization. *Journal of Consulting and Clinical Psychology*, 1965, *29*, 1–8.

Castaneda, A., McCandless, B. R., & Palermo, D. S. The children's form of the Manifest Anxiety Scale. *Child Development*, 1956, *27*, 317–326.

Cataldo, M. F., Bessman, G. A., Parker, L. H., Pearson, J. E. R., & Rogers, M. C. Behavioral assessment for pediatric intensive care units. *Journal of Applied Behavior Analysis*, 1979, *12*, 83–97.

Cataldo, M. F., Jacobs, H. E., & Rogers, M. C. Behavioral/environmental considerations in pediatric inpatient care. In D. C. Russo & J. W. Varni (eds.),

Behavioral pediatrics: Research and practice. New York: Plenum Press, in press.

Cataldo, M. F., & Risley, T. R. Evaluation of living environments: The MAN-IFEST description of ward activities. In P. O. Davison, F. W. Clark, & L. A. Hamerlynck (eds.), *Evaluation of behavioral programs in community residential and school settings*. Champaign, Ill.: Research Press, 1974, 201–222.

Chapman, A. H., Loeb, D. G., & Gibbons, M. J. Psychiatric aspects of hospitalizing children. *Archives of Pediatrics*, 1956, *73*, 77–88.

Cuthbertson, D. P. The disturbance of metabolism produced by bony and non-bony injury, with notes of certain abnormal conditions of bone. *Biochemical Journal*, 1930, *24*, 1244–1263.

Egerton, N., & Kay, J. H. Psychological disturbances associated with open heart surgery. *British Journal of Psychiatry*, 1964, *110*, 433–439.

Fagin, C. M. The case of rooming in when young children are hospitalized. *Nursing Science*, 1964, *2*, 324.

Ferguson, B. F. Preparing young children for hospitalization: A comparison of two methods. *Pediatrics*, 1979, *64*, 656–664.

Fishman, J. R., Hamburg, D. A., Handlon, J. H., Mason, J. W., & Sachar, E. Emotional and adrenal cortical responses to a new experience. *Archives of General Psychiatry*, 1962, *6*, 29–36.

Forsyth R. P. Blood pressure responses to long-term avoidance schedules in the restrained rhesus monkey. *Psychosomatic Medicine*, 1969, *31*, 300–309.

Friedman, S. B., Ader, R., & Glasgow, L. A. Effect of psychological stress in adult mice innoculated with Coxsakie B virus. *Psychosomatic Medicine*, 1965, *27*, 361–368.

Gann, D. S. Endocrine control of plasma protein and volume. *Surgical Clinics of North America*, 1976, *56*, 1135–1145.

Gellert, E. Reducing the emotional stresses of hospitalization for children. *American Journal of Occupational Therapy*, 1958, *12*:3, 125–129.

Glazer, H. I., Weiss, J. M., Pohorecky, L. A., & Miller, N. E. Monoamines as mediators of avoidance–escape behavior. *Psychosomatic Medicine*, 1975, *37*, 535–543.

Haller, J. A., Talbert, J. L., & Dombro, R. H. *The hospitalized child and his family*. Baltimore: Johns Hopkins University Press, 1967.

Harrison, T. S., Seaton, J. F., & Feller, I. Relationship of increased oxygen consumption to catecholamine excretion in thermal burns. *Annals of Surgery*, 1967, *165*, 169–172.

Herd, J. A., Morse, W. H., Kelleher, R. T., & Jones, L. G. Arterial hypertension in the squirrel monkey during behavioral experiments. *American Journal of Physiology*, 1969, *217*, 25–29.

Jackson, K., Winkley, R., Faust, O. A., Cermak, E. G., & Burtt, M. M. Behavior changes indicating emotional trauma in tonsillectomized children. *Pediatrics*, 1953, *12*, 23–27.

Jarhult, J. Osmotic fluid transfer from tissue to blood during hemorrhagic hypotension. *Acta Physiologica Scandinavica*, 1973, *89*, 213.

Jarhult, J., Lundvall, J., Mellander, S. & Tibblin S. Osmolar control of plasma volume during hemorrhagic hypotension. *Acta Physiologica Scandinavica,* 1972, *85,* 142.

Jessner, L., Blom, G. E., & Waldfogel, S. Emotional implications of tonsillectomy and adenoidectomy in children. In R. S. Eissler, A. Freud, H. Hartmann, & E. Kris (eds.), *The psychoanalytic study of the child.* New York: International al Universities Press, 1952.

Kagan, A., & Levi, L. Health and environment—Psychosocial stimuli: A review. In L. Levi (ed.), *Society, stress and disease. Vol. 2: Childhood and Adolescence.* London: Oxford University Press, 1975.

Katz, E. R., Kellerman, J., & Siegel, S. E. Behavioral distress in children with cancer undergoing medical procedures: Developmental considerations. *Journal of Consulting and Clinical Psychology,* 1980, *48,* 356–365.

Klinedinst, J. K. Multiphasic measures of child personality: Construction of content scales using the Personality Inventory for Children. *Journal of Consulting and Clinical Psychology,* 1975, *43*:5, 708–715.

Koppitz, E. M. *Psychological evaluation of children's human figure drawings.* New York: Grune & Stratton, 1968.

Kornfeld, D. S. The hospital environment: Its impact on the patient. In R. H. Moos (ed.), *Coping with physical illness.* New York: Plenum Medical Book Company, 1977.

Kornfeld, D. S., Zimberg, S., & Malm, J. R. Psychiatric complications of open-heart surgery. *New England Journal of Medicine,* 1965, *273,* 287–292.

Lawson, K., Daum, C., & Turkewitz, G. Environmental characteristics of a neonatal intensive-care unit. *Child Development,* 1977, *48,* 1633–1639.

Lazarus, H. R., & Hagens, J. H. Prevention of psychosis following open-heart surgery. *American Journal of Psychiatry,* 1968, *124,* 1190–1195.

Lazarus, R. S. Stress. In D. L. Sills (ed.), *The International Encyclopedia of the Social Sciences.* Vol. 15. New York: Macmillan, 1968.

Margetts, E. L. Historical notes on psychosomatic medicine. In E. D. Wittkower & R. A. Cleghorn (eds.), *Recent developments in psychosomatic medicine.* Philadelphia: Lippincott, 1954.

Mason, J. W., Sachar, E. J., Fishman, J. R., Hamburg, D. A., & Handlon, J. H. Corticosteroid responses to hospital admission. *Archives of General Psychiatry,* 1965, *13,* 1–8.

McKegney, F. P. The intensive care syndrome. *Connecticut Medicine,* 1966, *30,* 633–636.

Melamed, B. G., & Siegel, L. J. Reduction of anxiety in children facing hospitalization and surgery by use of filmed modeling. *Journal of Consulting and Clinical Psychology,* 1975, *43,* 511–521.

Miller, S. M. When is a little information a dangerous thing? Coping with stressful events by monitoring vs. blunting. In S. Levine & H. Ursin (eds.), *Coping and health.* New York: Plenum Press, 1980.

Miller, W., & Seligman, M. E. P. Depression and the perception of reinforcement. *Journal of Abnormal Psychology,* 1973, *9,* 62–73.

Moot, S. A., Cebulla, R. P., & Crabtree, J. M. Instrumental control and ulceration in rats. *Journal of Comparative Physiological Psychology*, 1970, 71, 405–410.

Nagera, H. Children's reactions to hospitalization and illness, *Child Psychiatry and Human Development*, 1978, 9, 3–19.

Nelson, G. N., Masuda, M., & Holmes, T. H. Correlation of behavior and catecholamine metabolite excretion. *Psychosomatic Medicine*, 1966, 28, 216–222.

Pavlov, I. P. *Conditioned reflexes*. New York: Dover, 1927.

Pearson, J. E. R., Cataldo, M., Tureman, A., Bessman, C., & Rogers, M. C. Pediatric intensive care unit patients: Effects of play intervention on behavior. *Critical Care Medicine*, 1980, 8:2, 64–67.

Persky, H., Korchin, S. J., Basowitz, H., Board, F. A., Sabshin, M., Hamburg, D., & Grinker, R. R. Effect of two psychological stresses on adrenocortical function. *Archives of Neurology and Psychiatry*, 1959, 81, 219–226.

Peterson, L., & Ridley-Johnson, R. Pediatric hospital response to survey on prehospital preparation for children. *Journal of Pediatric Psychology*, 1980, 5, 1–7.

Pirkle, J. C., & Gann, D. S. Restitution of blood volume after hemorrhage: Role of the adrenal cortex. *American Journal of Physiology*, 1976, 230, 1683–1687.

Price, D. B., Thaler, M., & Mason, J. W. Pre-operative emotional states and adrenal cortical activity. *Archives of Neurology and Psychiatry*, 1957, 77, 646–656.

Prugh, D., Staub, E., Sands, H., Kirschbaum, R., & Lenihan, E. A study of the emotional reactions of children and families to hospitalization and illness. *American Journal of Orthopsychiatry*, 1953, 23, 70–106.

Reim, B., Glass, D. C., & Singer, J. E. Behavioral consequences of exposure to uncontrollable and unpredictable noise. *Journal of Applied Social Psychology*, 1971, 1, 44–56.

Rescorla, R. A., & LoLordo, V. M. Inhibition of avoidance behavior. *Journal of Comparative and Physiological Psychology*, 1965, 59, 406–412.

Rie, H. E., Boverman, H., Grossman, B. J., & Ozoa, N. Immediate and long-term effects of interventions early in prolonged hospitalization. *Pediatrics*, 1968, 41, 755–764.

Rubin, R. T., & Mandell, A. J. Adrenal cortical activity in pathological emotional states: A review. *American Journal of Psychiatry*, 1966, 123, 387–400.

Schaffer, H. R. Objective observations of personality development in early infancy. *British Journal of Medical Psychology*, 1958, 31, 174–183.

Schaffer, J. R., & Callender, W. H. Psychological effects of hospitalization in infancy. *Pediatrics*, 1959, 24, 528–539.

Scherer, M. W., & Nakamura, C. Y. A fear survey schedule for children (FSS-FC): A factor analytic comparison with manifest anxiety (CMAS). *Behaviour Research and Therapy*, 1968, 6, 173–182.

Seligman, M. E. *Helplessness: On depression, development and death*. San Francisco: W. H. Freeman, 1975.

Selye, H. *The stress of life*. New York: McGraw-Hill, 1976.

Shorkey, C. T., & Taylor, J. E. Management of maladaptive behavior of a severely burned child. *Child Welfare*, 1973, *52*, 543–547.

Sidman, M. Time-out from avoidance as a reinforcer: A study of response interaction. *Journal of the Experimental Analysis of Behavior*, 1962, *5*, 423–434.

Skipper, J. K., & Leonard, R. C. Children, stress and hospitalization: A field experiment. *Journal of Health and Social Behavior*, 1968, *9*, 275–287.

Toch, H. H., & Hastorf, A. H. Homeostasis in psychology, a review and critique. *Psychiatry*, 1955, *18*, 81–91.

Ulvedal, F., Smith, W. R., & Welch, B. E. Steroid and catecholamine studies on pilots during prolonged experiments in a space cabin simulator. *Journal of Applied Physiology*, 1963, *18*, 1257.

Vaughan, G. F. Children in hospital. *Lancet*, 1957, *272*, 1117–1120.

Vernon, D., Foley, J., & Schulman, J. Effect of mother–child separation and birth order on young children's responses to two potentially stressful experiences. *Journal of Personality and Social Psychology*, 1967, *5*, 423–434.

Vernon, D., Foley, J., Sipowicz, R., & Schulman, J. *The psychological responses of children to hospitalization and illness. A review of the literature*. Springfield, Illinois: Charles C Thomas, 1965.

Vernon, D., Schulman, J., & Foley, J. Changes in children's behavior after hospitalization. *American Journal of Diseases of Children*, 1966, *111*, 581–593.

Visintainer, M., & Wolfer, J. Psychological preparation for surgical pediatric patients: The effect on children's and parents' stress responses and adjustment. *Pediatrics*, 1975, *56*, 187–202.

Weiss, J. M. Effects of coping behavior in different warning signal conditions on stress pathology in rats. *Journal of Comparative Physiological Psychology*, 1971, *77*, 1–13.

Weiss, J. M., Glazer, H. I., & Pohorecky, L. A. Coping behavior and neurochemical changes: An alternative explanation for the original "learned helplessness" experiments. In G. Serban & A. Kling (eds.), *Animal models in human psycho-biology*. New York: Plenum, 1976.

Weiss, J. M., Glazer, H. I., Pohorecky, L. A., Brick, J., & Miller, N. E. Effects of chronic exposure to stressors on avoidance–escape behavior and on brain norepinephrine. *Psychosomatic Medicine*, 1975, *37*, 522–534.

Weiss, J. M., Stone, E. A., & Harrell, N. Coping behavior and brain norepinephrine level in rats. *Journal of Comparative and Physiological Psychology*, 1970, *72*, 153–160.

Weissman, R. G., & Litner, J. S. Role of the inter-trial interval in Pavlovian differential conditioning of fear in rats. *Journal of Comparative and Physiological Psychology*, 1971, *74*, 211–218.

Wilmore, D. W., Long, J. M., Mason, A. D., Skreen, R. W., and Pruitt, B. A. Catecholamines: Mediator of the hypermetabolic response to thermal injury. *Annals of Surgery*, 1974, *180*, 653–669.

Wolfer, J. A., & Visintainer, M. A. Prehospital psychological preparation for tonsillectomy patients—Effect on children's and parent's adjustment. *Pediatrics*, 1979, *64*, 646–655.

CHAPTER 6

Cigarette Smoking: Why Young People Do It and Ways of Preventing It

Brian R. Flay, D. Phil.
Josie R. d'Avernas, M.Sc.
J. Allan Best, Ph.D.
Mary W. Kersell, M.Sc.
Katherine B. Ryan, B.A.

Introduction

Four reports by the U.S. Surgeon General (U.S. Public Health Service, 1964, 1979, 1980, 1981) illustrate the wide-ranging influence that smoking can have on health, including an increased risk for heart disease, lung cancer, chronic bronchitis, peptic ulcer, respiratory disorders, damage and injuries due to fires and accidents, lower birth weight, and retarded fetal development.

The evidence linking smoking to poor health has sparked considerable research in the area of smoking cessation. Hundreds of cessation programs have been designed and evaluated; however, although the majority of procedures are capable of producing short-term behavioral change, high rates of relapse are almost universal. Thus, recent reviews (Bernstein &

The research reported here was supported by Ontario Ministry of Health Grant #CHS-R26. Brian R. Flay was partially supported by NIDA grant #5 R01 DA 02941 02 (C. A. Johnson, principal investigator) while writing this chapter. We wish to thank K. Stephen Brown for guidance in data analysis and William B. Hansen, Karen M. Hennigan, and C. Anderson Johnson for helpful comments.

McAlister, 1976; Best & Bloch, 1979; Lichtenstein & Danaher, 1976; Pechacek, 1979) have concluded that the wide range of smoking cessation techniques usually are ineffective, at least in the long term. Although it is premature to reject cessation as a strategy for controlling smoking, an alternative approach—such as prevention—needs to be developed and evaluated.

Several indications support the importance of a preventative approach in dealing with the problem of smoking in youth. The probability of regular smoking in childhood leading to a lifetime of smoking and the consequent increases in morbidity and mortality is high (Salber, Freeman, & Abelin, 1968). Smoking also has been linked with respiratory disorders in children. This association comes both from self-reports of children (Bewley & Bland, 1976; Bewley, Halil, & Snaith, 1973; Cameron, 1972; Rush, 1974; Stanhope & Prior, 1975) and from clinical studies (Harrison, Mohler, Lewis, & Speir, 1979). The possibility of delaying onset in itself may be advantageous. For example, a study summarized in the 1979 Surgeon General's report indicates that the mortality of those who smoked since they were 15 years old was 50 percent higher than those who started smoking in their twenties. The prevalence of smoking in younger children has increased in recent years, as the age of onset has decreased (Brown, Cherry, & Forbes, 1978; Health and Welfare Canada, 1977, 1979; U.S. Public Health Service, 1979). This suggests increasing health problems in future generations. Finally, recent social psychologically based smoking prevention programs appear to have been effective in preventing or delaying the onset of regular smoking in adolescents (Botvin, Eng, & Williams, 1980; Evans, Rozelle, Mittelmark, Hansen, Bane, & Havis, 1978; Hurd, Johnson, Pechacek, Bast, Jacobs, & Luepker, 1980; McAlister, Perry, Killen, Slinkard, & Maccoby, 1980).

We have four main goals in this chapter. The first is to review the literature on the process of becoming a smoker and to use this information to derive a new developmental causal model of the process of becoming a smoker. The second goal is to review school-based attempts to prevent adolescents from becoming smokers. Two major types of interventions will be reviewed: (1) traditional educational programs that rely almost completely on disseminating information and (2) newer programs, based on social psychological theories, which attempt to provide adolescents with decision-making and social skills to help them resist the pressures to become smokers. The third goal is to provide herein the first published description of our own study at the University of Waterloo and to report some of the recently obtained results. The fourth and final goal is to integrate our knowledge of the antecedents of smoking, our new model of the process of becoming a smoker, and our knowledge of the effectiveness of various interventions, all in order to derive implications for future program development and research.

The Process of Becoming a Smoker

In this section we (1) present the stages invoked by past and current researchers to describe the process of becoming a smoker, (2) review current knowledge about the antecedents of smoking, and (3) combine these two sets of knowledge to derive a new developmental causal model of the process of becoming a cigarette smoker.

Stages of Smoking

Much of the literature on the development of smoking has not been very informative because either discussion of the problem has been focused too narrowly or research has been unsound methodologically. When considering youth, the question of why people smoke needs to be broken down into several issues that relate to the developmental history of smoking. Recent smoking prevention researchers have tended to recognize three stages: trying the first cigarette, experimental smoking (less than weekly), and regular smoking (at least weekly). Possibly as many as 90 percent of us have tried at least one cigarette at some time. By age 12, around 10 percent of teenagers already are smoking at least once a week. By age 15, this has increased to around 30 percent, and by age 18 it has reached 40 percent. Figure 6.1 illustrates the onset curve (Brown et al., 1978). Recent figures for the United States were slightly lower than these with a further slight decrease evident in later years (Green, 1979; Johnston, Bachman, & O'Malley, 1977, 1979). Among United States high-school seniors, the rate of daily smoking was still around 30 percent in the mid-1970s, but down around 20 percent by 1981 (Johnston, Bachman and O'Malley, 1982). At least 20 percent of adults are former smokers, indicating that at least 60 percent of young adults were regular smokers at some stage during their lives. The leveling off of the onset curve by high-school grades 10–12 suggests that most initiation and experimentation now is occurring during the junior high school years or before. The recent increase in the number of teenage girls smoking now seems to be leveling off at the same rate as boys (Brown et al., 1978; Johnston et al., 1982).

While the three behavioral stages of trying, experimenting, and smoking regularly provide convenient steps for measurement purposes, it is not clear that they describe adequately the development of smoking behavior. Earlier work, reviewed by Leventhal & Cleary (1980), led to the suggestion of a four-stage process: preparation, initiation, becoming a smoker,

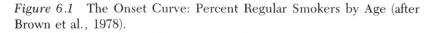

Figure 6.1 The Onset Curve: Percent Regular Smokers by Age (after Brown et al., 1978).

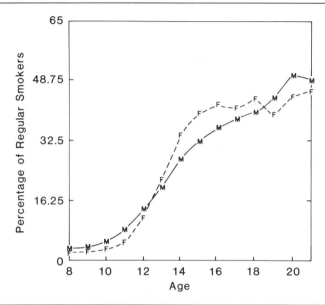

and maintenance of smoking. The major contribution here is the recognition of a preparation or anticipation stage. Clearly, a number of psychological, environmental, and possibly biological factors prepare certain youths to be smokers and certain others to remain nonsmokers. Another contribution of this model is the attempt to explain what processes are involved at each stage, rather than the simple description of each stage in behavioral terms.

The various models of the stages in the process of becoming a smoker are shown graphically in Figure 6.2 and may be summarized in the following way. Preparation and anticipation sometimes will lead to trying the first cigarette (initiation), which sometimes will be followed by repeated experimentation (learning), possibly sufficiently often (becoming) for the acquisition of a habit and for addictive processes to take hold (maintaining) (Pomerleau, 1979a, b). The process of becoming a smoker appears to be a stochastic one, with the probability of going from one stage to the next always less than one. Thus, we all had the option of remaining neversmokers, although most of us have tried cigarettes at least once. Similarly, having tried one cigarette, we may decide never to try another or we may experiment further. Once at the experimenter stage, we may decide to

Figure 6.2 Stages in the Development of Smoking Behavior during
Adolescence.

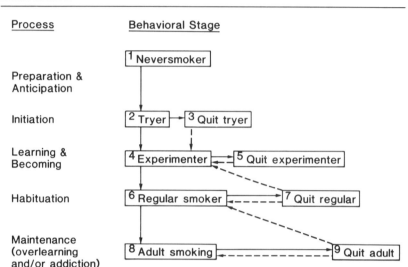

quit or continue experimenting sufficiently often to become a regular
smoker. Up to 1968, between 70 percent and 90 percent of teenagers who
tried four or more cigarettes became regular smokers (McKennel & Thomas, 1967; Salber et al., 1968). Becoming a regular smoker as an adolescent
(i.e., at least weekly), does not, of course, necessarily mean becoming a
habitual smoker as an adult. At least one-third of those adults who currently do not smoke did so at some point in their lives. Alternatively, quitting at
any stage need not be a final decision. There is always the possibility of
returning to the last or a previous stage of smoking.

We now will review the available literature on the antecedents of
smoking by youth. Following that, we will develop a more detailed developmental model of the process of becoming a smoker.

Antecedents of Smoking by Youth

Research on the antecedents of smoking has been voluminous; however,
most studies have been cross-sectional or retrospective in nature, so that
causal inferences cannot be drawn. In addition, no studies reported to date
have attempted to determine the different antecedents for the different
stages of the process of becoming a smoker. Rather, they have simply
attempted to discriminate smokers from nonsmokers.

The factors most investigated as correlates of smoking behavior will be reviewed in these five categories: social, sociodemographic, personality, psychosocial, and biological.

Social Factors. Early smoking frequently has been blamed on *social factors*, such as early exposure to a smoking environment (Baric, 1979). Parental smoking behavior and attitudes and peer smoking both have been found to be highly associated with adolescent smoking. These factors often vie for the primary predictive position (Allegrante, O'Rourke, & Tuncalp, 1977; Bewley, Bland, & Harris, 1974; Borland, 1975; Bynner, 1969; Chassin, Presson, Bensenberg, Corty, Olshavsky, & Sherman, 1981; Gritz & Brunswick, 1980; Hranchuk, Christie, Hranchuk, & Kennedy, 1978; Kelson, Pullella, & Otterland, 1975; Levitt & Edwards, 1970; McKennel, 1970; Newman, 1970a, 1970b; Newman, Martin, & Irwin, 1973; Palmer, 1970; Pederson & Lefcoe, in press; Pederson, Baskerville, & Lefcoe, 1981a, b; Salber, Welsh, & Taylor, 1963; Williams, 1971). Some studies have suggested that parents' approval or disapproval of their children's smoking may be particularly important if these attitudes are consistent with the parents' own behavior (Allegrante et al., 1977; Kelson et al., 1975; Palmer, 1970). The social influence of same-sex family members or peers seems to be especially important (Kelson et al., 1975). The total number of smokers in a young person's environment is also influential, with more smokers increasing the probability of subsequent smoking by the youngster (Bewley et al., 1974; Glasgow, McCaul, O'Neil, Freeborn, & Spreier, 1981; U.S. Public Health Service, 1976).

Data about the occasion for the first cigarette also show the social nature of smoking. Over 50 percent of adolescents report smoking their first cigarette with a friend (Bewley et al., 1974; Palmer, 1970). Only 16 percent of boys and nine percent of girls report smoking their first cigarette alone. A surprising five percent of boys and two percent of girls report having their first cigarette with a parent (Palmer, 1970).

The effects of mass media and advertising, which associate smoking with fun, risk taking, sexual adventure, and maturity, also are thought to be significant social influences on smoking behavior (Goldberg & Gorn, 1978; Gorn & Goldberg, 1977a, b; Gritz & Brunswick, 1980; Moser, 1974). However, there is as yet no persuasive empirical evidence that the media influence the decision to start smoking (Fishbein, 1977; McAlister, Perry, & Maccoby, 1979; Mettlin, 1976; Kelson et al., 1975). It seems likely, though, that all media contribute indirectly to social pressure by supporting the use of cigarettes as a sign of maturity and autonomy (Dekker, 1977; McAlister et al., 1979).

Sociodemographic Variables. These include socioeconomic status, sex, and performance in school. There is a consistent, though not always strong, negative association between socioeconomic status and smoking, particularly among boys (Borland, 1975; Kozlowski, 1979a, b; McKennel & Thomas, 1967; Salber & McMahon, 1961). This relationship is less evident and may even be reversed for girls. If the increased smoking among girls is due to changing sex roles and the accompanying pressures, we might even expect a positive association in the future, rather than a negative one (Gritz, 1977; Schuman, 1977).

Low academic goals and performance have been associated consistently with smoking among adolescents (Bewley & Bland, 1976; Borland, 1975; Creswell, Huffman, & Stone, 1970; Horn, 1963; Hranchuk et al., 1978; Jessor & Jessor, 1977; Laoye, Creswell, & Stone, 1972; Newman, 1970b). Smoking teenagers also have been found to be doing less well in meeting other expectations of parents and traditional authorities (Newman, 1970a; Smith, 1970; Stewart & Livson, 1966).

Personality. Hundreds of studies have attempted to establish associations between personality variables and smoking. Unfortunately, most have been done with adults and so might be more likely to relate to the maintenance of smoking than to its establishment. We cannot assume that a personality characteristic associated with smoking in adulthood even was present in adolescence, let alone predictive of subsequent behavior. It even is possible that regular smoking influences personality.

The available studies on adolescents (e.g., Cherry & Kiernan, 1976; Clausen, 1968; Coan, 1973; McKennel & Thomas, 1967; Reynolds & Nichols, 1976; Smith, 1969; Williams, 1971) have found few personality variables that discriminate consistently between adolescents who will begin to smoke regularly and those who will remain nonsmokers. A large, longitudinal study (Cherry & Kiernan, 1976) showed that extroversion and neuroticism each were associated positively with becoming a smoker for both sexes. The finding for extroversion has been replicated by Reynolds & Nichols (1976) and Smith (1969), each of whom also found other correlates of smoking related to overall adjustment. It is probable that smoking onset may be affected by some personality factors; however, the specific mechanisms by which these operate are unclear. Recent data on self-image might offer a possible explanation (Chassin, Presson, Sherman, Corty, & Olshavsky, 1981).

Psychosocial Variables. These are concerned with the interaction of internal variables, such as personality traits, and external variables, such as social influences. They are concerned with how certain types of individuals react to certain types of situations. Such variables may come closer to providing a phenomenological description of why people in general smoke and why adolescents in particular start to smoke.

Several authors (Jessor & Jessor, 1977; Russell, 1977) have noted that many adolescents, especially those not performing well in school, adopt adult behaviors, such as taking a job, drinking alcohol, smoking cigarettes, and engaging in sexual intercourse. Teenagers who smoke cigarettes and drink beer are also more likely to go on to try marijuana and harder drugs (Gould, Berberian, Kasl, Thompson, & Kleber, 1977; Jessor, 1976, 1978; Johnson, Graham, & Hansen, 1981; Kandel, 1975, 1978; Seltzer, Friedman, & Siegelaub, 1974; Tennant & Detels, 1976). These findings suggest that an important incentive for the adolescent smoker might be the desire for accelerated maturity. Evans and his colleagues (Evans, Henderson, Hill, & Raines, 1979) found that looking more mature was one of the major benefits of smoking, as perceived by adolescents. Other explanations for the association of these behaviors are possible, however; it may simply be that those behaviors are associated with large amounts of spare time for risk taking. Other perceived benefits reported by Evans et al. (1979) were appearing tougher, more sociable, and more like a leader. These suggest that smoking might be a substitute for other social reinforcers.

McKennel & Thomas (1967) identified two broad categories of motives for smoking perceived by smoking and nonsmoking teenagers as well as adults. One category consisted of inner need factors such as nervous irritation, relaxation, smoking alone, activity accompaniment, and food substitution. The second category consisted of social factors such as social smoking and social-confidence smoking. A remarkably similar set of factors, with the addition of an "addiction" factor, was derived by Tomkins (1966) and replicated on several samples by Leventhal & Avis (1976).

McKennel & Thomas (1967) also stratified their sample of teenagers according to stage of smoking, so that some of their findings are especially relevant to a model of the development of smoking. Social smoking increased steadily during adolescence and then declined during adult life. Social-confidence smoking decreased during adult life, with the biggest drop occurring after the first two or three years of smoking. There was a rapid increase in nervous-irritation smoking during the first two years of regular smoking, suggesting that it might take about two years to become dependent. Adolescents were slightly ahead of adults on most inner-need factors, as well as activity accompaniment; that is, it seems that smoking helped to satisfy inner needs very soon after smoking was started. While this study requires cautious interpretation because of (1) its cross-sectional nature and (2) the confounding of prevalence of smoking with reason for smoking, these findings are suggestive and will be incorporated into our developmental model of the process of becoming a smoker. Knowledge and beliefs about smoking and smokers, attitudes toward them, and behavioral intentions regarding them often are thought to be predictive, if not causative, of subsequent smoking (Fishbein, 1977; Fishbein & Ajzen, 1975). Most studies of the relationship among knowledge, beliefs, attitudes, and intentions about smoking have been cross-sectional or retrospective, making causal inference hazardous at best. Consistently, however, smoking adolescents have less knowledge about the negative consequences of smoking and have fewer negative beliefs about and attitudes toward smoking than their nonsmoking counterparts (Beaglehole, Eyles, & Harding, 1978; Bewley et al., 1974, Brown et al., 1978; Canadian Home and School, 1973; Hranchuk et al., 1978; Kelson et al., 1975; Newman et al., 1973; Pederson & Lefcoe, in press; Pederson et al., 1981a, b; Schneider & Van Mastrigt, 1974). In at least two studies (Green, 1979; Newman, Martin, & Peterson, 1978, cited in Leventhal & Cleary, 1980), a statement of intentions to try cigarettes was the best single predictor of later smoking. Data from prospective studies (Downey & O'Rourke, 1976; Glasgow et al., 1981) support the view that attitudes may have a causative influence on smoking behavior.

While smokers differ from nonsmokers in their knowledge, beliefs, and attitudes regarding smoking, most teenagers in both groups do in fact have high levels of knowledge and awareness of the negative health consequences of smoking. Even by grade 6, children can differentiate short-term and long-term consequences of smoking and already evidence some feelings of susceptibility to these consequences (Hansen & Mittlemark, 1981). Young people not yet smoking, however, seem to be unaware of the problem of addiction or dependence, believing instead that if they start smoking they will be able to stop whenever they want (Brecher, 1972).

Interacting with young people's knowledge, beliefs, attitudes, and intentions are their perceptions of the social support for smoking. Some theories, such as Fishbein & Ajzen (1975), would suggest that such perceptions play an important role in determining behavior (Schneider & Van Mastrigt, 1974). It seems that youth's perception of their social environment is biased in such a way that they perceive smoking as more common than it actually is. The American Cancer Society (1976) reported that 83 percent of adolescents see most teenagers as smoking, when only about 15 percent to 30 percent actually do. Two-thirds of teenagers also judge most teachers to be smokers (Jarvik, Cullen, Gritz, Vogt, & West, 1977), whereas the American Cancer Society (1976) found that only about 20 percent of teachers actually smoke. Some prospective studies have found that both attitudes and normative beliefs had significant and powerful effects on smoking (Chassin, Presson, Sherman, et al., 1981; Johnson, Murray, Jacobs, Pechacek, Hurd, & Luepker, 1979).

It is apparent from the literature that teenagers' knowledge and beliefs about, attitudes toward, and intentions regarding smoking are related to their actual smoking behavior. There is very little evidence, however, that these relationships are causal, although the few prospective studies available do tend to support this hypothesis.

Biological Factors. Those that can be implicated in the establishment of the smoking habit have not been thoroughly investigated yet. However, many of the immediate physiological and pharmacological effects of a first cigarette are known, and some of these are thought to deter some youths from further experimentation while encouraging others to continue experimenting. The initial harshness of smoking may be a critical factor influencing many to never try again. For others, however, the initial harshness may represent a challenge to be overcome (Leventhal, Brown, Shacham, & Engquist, 1979; Leventhal & Everhart, 1979). Jarvik and colleagues (Jarvik, 1979; Jarvik & Wong-McCarthy, in press) have reviewed the literature on pharmacological reinforcers of cigarettes that may facilitate the establishment of the smoking habit. They found that out of 36 possible contenders, nicotine appears to be the most responsible. Nicotine readily crosses the blood–brain barrier (Oldendorf, 1977) and has almost immediate effects on the central nervous system, the most important of which appears to be modulation of arousal levels (Itil, Ulett, Hsu, Klingenberg, & Ulett, 1971; Kales, Allen, Preston, Tan, & Kales, 1970; Ulett & Itil, 1969). Other pharmacological effects are the release of certain catecholamines (Jarvik, 1979) that are thought to produce a number of effects on the cardiovascular system. These have been summarized in the Surgeon General's reports (U.S. Public Health Service, 1979) and include increases in heart rate, blood pressure, and cardiac output. These effects occur in both nonsmokers and smokers after smoking one or two cigarettes. There are, as yet, no controlled experiments that adequately investigate nicotine's effects on the cardiovascular system as contributors to the reinforcing properties of cigarettes (Jarvik, 1979).

Other short-term effects of smoking include smelly breath and clothes, yellowing of the teeth and fingers, and decreased athletic performance. When made salient to youth, these effects may deter regular smoking.

The Maintenance of Smoking

The factors that are thought to explain why people continue to smoke have been reviewed numerous times. They include biological, biochemical, and physiological reactions (Jarvik, 1979), as well as psychological and psychosocial factors (Kozlowski, 1979a, b). These will not be reviewed in detail, since our focus is on the establishment of the behavior, not its maintenance. We simply note that smoking is an overlearned habit (Pomerleau, 1979a, b) and that for some people it also is dependence producing (Jarvik, 1979; Schacter, 1978). Leventhal & Cleary (1980) review and integrate the biological and psychosocial factors of the maintenance of smoking into a "multiple regulation" model.

A New Developmental–Causal Model of the
Process of Becoming a Smoker

We have suggested already (see Figure 6.2) that the establishment of smoking during adolescence may occur in several stages in a developmental sequence. The most important of these for adolescents are the preparation, initiation, experimentation, and becoming stages. In this section we shall use the findings about the antecedents of smoking, presented previously, to derive a more detailed model.

1.   *Preparation.* The preparation stage consists largely of the early learning experiences provided in a child's environment. A young child first becomes conscious of cigarettes as early as four months, and by three years over 90 percent of children are familiar with cigarettes (Baric & Fischer, 1979).

It is an obvious truism that smoking parents often provide the first model of the "adult behavior" of smoking. Smokers in the family are likely to have the primary influence in transferring the smoking habit to other family members because they have the longest contact with their family. On the other hand, smoking by peers also may be an important influence because peer recognition and approval become more important in adolescence (Erikson, 1963). We suspect that family influences are most important in the preparation stage, providing the vicarious experiences that allow for the development of attitudes about smoking, images of what smoking is like and why it is done, and intentions to try cigarettes (Leventhal & Cleary, 1980). Children view smoking as socially acceptable adult behavior, despite parental and medical advice against it. Smoking by family members, whether parents or siblings, also may provide the environment and materials for first trying a cigarette.

2.   *Initiation.* For most first-time smokers however, peer influences are probably more important than family influences in determining when cigarettes are first tried. We say when, rather than whether, because 80 percent to 90 percent of all teenagers have tried smoking at least once (Grant & Weitman, 1968; Palmer, 1970; Wohlford & Giammona, 1969). But exactly what are these peer influences? Some teenagers may feel anxious and inadequate, so they smoke to achieve social acceptance. Wong-McCarthy (1980) has hypothesized that this is a likely explanation for those youths trying their first cigarette at a stage of social transition such as the changes from grade school to junior high school or from junior high to high school. Much first-time smoking is thought to occur shortly after such transitions (Bergin & Wake, 1974; Horn, Courts, Taylor, & Solomon, 1959; Salber, Goldman, & Welsh, 1961). Other youths may try their first cigarette as only one of many experimental activities they share with a close

friend. Still others, particularly those who do not start until relatively late in adolescence, may start smoking to control such emotions as work or examination anxiety (Smith, 1970).

Children who are less successful in school or at meeting expectations of authority figures may be attracted to using cigarettes as a means of overcoming the resulting low self-image of themselves (Dekker, 1977; Gritz, 1977; Hasenfus, 1971; Huntwork & Ferguson, 1977; Mausner, 1973; Palmer, 1970; Salber, Welsh, & Taylor, 1963) or as a means of defining themselves as tough, cool, and independent of authority. This factor, improving one's self-image, is not necessarily different from seeking social approval, but it can be. Improving one's self-image can be motivated by poor performance in school and poor performance in the eyes of adults, as well as by low approval from desired peer groups.

3.　*Experimentation*. Once the first cigarette has been tried, the experimentation stage may begin. Whether or not it does will depend to some extent on the experience of that first cigarette. For some, the harshness of the first cigarette will put them off ever trying another. For others, however, the initial harshness simply will be something to be overcome. Some first-time smokers might have a very positive experience, obtaining positive reinforcement from increased heart rate and the other biological changes that occur, or from increased peer approval.

Family smoking may continue to operate as an influence at the experimentation stage, particularly by increasing the opportunities for obtaining cigarettes for experimentation (Baer & Katkin, 1971). The experimentation stage is one of learning: learning how to handle the cigarette, learning how to inhale correctly, and learning what the different effects are under different conditions. It is during this stage that reinforcers, both primary and secondary, both social and physiological, are experienced and conditioned.

4.　*Becoming*. If experimenting continues long enough, the transition will be made to regular smoking. Relatively old data suggest that about 85 percent to 90 percent of those who experiment with four or more cigarettes become regular smokers, and that the transition from first trying a cigarette to becoming a regular smoker can take up to two years (Salber et al., 1968).

It is during the stage of experimentation and the early stages of regular smoking, we believe, that the physiological effects have their greatest consequences. Initially, there are the immediate effects of stimulation of the nervous system and increased heart rate. It is probably through the repeated pairing of smoking with social and physiological reinforcement that the behavior becomes habitual. For some people at least, the habit becomes addictive, with the negative reinforcement of withdrawal symptoms adding to the positive reinforcement to continue smoking (Leventhal & Cleary, 1981).

Figure 6.3   A Preliminary Causal Model of the Major Influences, and Their Relative Strengths, on Stages of Smoking Behavior.

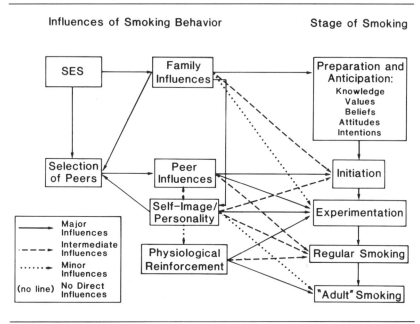

In Figure 6.3 we show a preliminary causal model of the major influences on the various stages of smoking behavior. A solid line indicates a major influence, a dashed line an intermediate influence, a dotted line a minor influence, while no line indicates no direct influence. To summarize, family influences appear to be most important during the preparation stage, having decreasing influence as the behavior develops. Peer pressures and problems with self-image or social competence take over as the major influences at the initiation stage. Attitudes formed during the preparation stage influence the selection of important peers. Most people select friends with similar attitudes. The choice of peers, of course, is limited by the child's environment, which is determined partly by his socioeconomic status. While socioeconomic status has been shown consistently to be correlated with smoking by males, we do not believe it has a direct influence; instead, we think it has an indirect effect by influencing whether or not a child's parents smoke and by influencing the child's selection of peers. At the stage of experimentation, peer pressure is still an important factor, but it is moderated by other social motives for smoking and perceptions of the physiological effects of the first few cigarettes. Both the social motives for smoking and perceptions of the physiological effects may be determined partially by personality factors, with social motives also being determined partially by peer influences. The social reinforcements obtained from smoking are probably the most important influence on whether or not an experimenting adolescent will become a regular smoker. Peer pressure still may play a role at this stage, although its effects probably are mediated through social reinforcement. Physiological effects also may be important at this stage, particularly for certain types of individuals. Changes in the pattern of smoking as an adolescent becomes an adult probably are influenced more and more by the physiological effects on emotional states, and less and less by social factors.

The model proposed here has several important implications. First, it helps integrate a previously unorganized mass of findings on the antecedents of smoking. Second, it may help explain some of the inconsistencies in that literature. For example, it may explain why some studies find family influences most predictive of smoking while other studies find peer influences most predictive. The present model suggests that each can be of prime importance, but at different stages in the process of becoming a smoker (Utech & Hoving, 1969). A third advantage of this model is that it considers adolescent development more than have other models of smoking onset. Obviously, youngsters of different ages perceive and experience their environment in different ways, and this model allows these changes to be incorporated. Fourth, this model is useful in providing causal hypotheses that can be tested. Some links could be tested by providing interventions (e.g., does improving students' social competence reduce the chances of their becoming smokers?). Most links, however, and the model as a whole, might best be tested first in prospective and longitudinal correlational studies, using the newer statistical techniques, such as LISREL, that involve structural modeling (Bentler, 1980; Jöreskog & Sörbom, 1978). Finally, this model has important implications for the design of interventions to prevent adolescents from becoming smokers. Before discussing these, we first will review the effectiveness of those interventions that have been tested to date.

School-Based Attempts to Prevent Smoking

Possible strategies for preventing adolescents from ever becoming regular smokers are many and varied. This review of prevention programs will be divided into three sections: first, traditional educational approaches will be reviewed; this will be followed by a detailed consideration of a number of recent social psychological approaches. The final section will be a report of our own psychosocial study, the Waterloo study.

Traditional Educational Approaches

Smoking-prevention studies include those reporting on school-based information campaigns, those comparing teaching methods, and those comparing message themes. Typically, school information campaigns, using a combination of discussions, lectures, demonstrations, assemblies, posters, pamphlets, films, articles in the school paper, and resource people to impart information on the dangers of smoking, have had no significant impact on smoking habits (Thompson, 1978). Evans (1979) suggested that, aside from methodological problems making evaluation of such campaigns almost impossible, teachers themselves often have expressed a lack of confidence in their ability to implement smoking-education programs effectively.

Since 1976, few school-based, antismoking programs have been reported in the literature. One that deserves mention as a promising approach is the School Health Curriculum Project (SHCP) (Heit, 1978; Iammarino, Heit, & Kaplan, 1980). SHCP uses a variety of approaches, designed for implementation from kindergarten through seventh grade, and is focused on health rather than on smoking specifically. A survey conducted with eighth-grade students, three years after participation in SHCP, indicated that they smoked significantly less than their counterparts who received either regular health education instruction or no health education instruction at all (Iammarino et al., 1980). While it cannot be said that SHCP alone accounted for these differences, the approach does seem promising.

Large-scale public information and prevention campaigns that are not solely school based also have failed to produce a significant impact on smoking (Bradshaw, 1973). Pointing to the many limitations of these campaigns, such as inadequate follow-up evaluations and failure to include comparison control groups, Bradshaw (1973) recommended a more systematic approach. Evans (1979) emphasized that these campaigns have been targeted too broadly and that they have not focused on children and adolescents, who should be the prime targets for such campaigns.

Thompson (1978) reported on several studies using or comparing various teacher-led programs, didactic approaches, group discussions, persuasion, presenting of one side versus both sides of the issue, encouragement of students to take an adult role, and use of media. No consistent effects were found.

At present, two areas of research regarding teaching methods are quite active. One is the area of peer-led programming. In these programs, junior or senior high-school students plan and carry out educational activities for their peers or for students in an earlier grade. One such program is the Saskatoon smoking study (Jones, Piper, & Mathews, 1970; Piper, Jones, &

Mathews, 1970, 1971, 1974), in which eighth-grade students from 32 schools attended a seminar on smoking and health and then returned to their respective schools to plan and execute smoking programs of their own. After two years, no significant difference existed between the smoking habits of students exposed to the peer-led program and those not exposed. The second area involves the use of media in smoking prevention, that is, the use of videotapes and films in programming. Both these strategies currently are being used, mainly with social psychological approaches to smoking prevention; they will be mentioned later.

Three main message themes have been reported in antismoking programming in the past (Thompson, 1978). The messages are (1) there are negative long-term effects of smoking on health, (2) there are negative short-term effects of smoking, and (3) the image of smokers is more negative than that of nonsmokers. Programs using the first theme have shown consistently negligible impact on behavior. Thompson (1978) reported some inconsistency in the results of studies comparing programs emphasizing immediate effects versus those emphasizing long-term effects of smoking. On the whole it appears that the immediate effects theme is more effective (Creswell, Huffman, Stone, Merki, & Newman, 1969; Creswell, Stone, Huffman, & Newman, 1971; Horn, 1960) or at least as effective as the long-term effects theme (Merki, Creswell, Stone, Huffman, & Newman, 1968). The third theme, comparing the image of smokers and nonsmokers, has been the subject of too little research to speculate on its effects.

In summary, traditional smoking-prevention programs generally have attempted to dissuade students from smoking by providing them with factual information on the dangers of smoking. The assumption has been that this information would influence beliefs, which in turn would lead to nonsmoking attitudes and subsequently to nonsmoking behavior. Of those programs that could be evaluated, many have succeeded in changing students' knowledge and attitudes about cigarette smoking, but they generally have not succeeded in preventing smoking onset.

Social Psychological Prevention Approaches

The failure of traditional smoking-prevention programs to consider social and psychological processes leading to the adoption of the smoking habit often has been blamed for the lack of success of these programs. The empirical literature on adolescent smoking suggests that onset is not caused by a single factor or event; rather, a combination of factors, including psychological and social, interact to influence initiation. Recently, more effort has gone into considering these complex psychological and social processes in the design of smoking-prevention strategies for adolescents. Richard Evans (1976) and his colleagues (Evans et al., 1978) developed and tested the first of a series of social psychologically based smoking-prevention programs targeted on smoking in early adolescence. The program incorporated a variety of psychological principles, including communications analysis (McGuire, 1969) and social inoculation (McGuire, 1964). Social inoculation is analagous to biological inoculation, whereby, in the latter, a person is exposed to a small dose of an infectious agent in order to develop antibodies, thereby reducing susceptibility to subsequent exposure. This model, applied to smoking, assumes that social factors exert the major influence on the initial decision to experiment with cigarettes. It further assumes that resistance to persuasion to smoke will be greater if one has developed, then refuted, arguments for smoking cigarettes in specific situations. According to the theory, such experience with counter-arguments inoculates the individual against pressures in similar real-life situations by developing resistance to these pressures in advance.

A program developed by Evans et al. (1978) used nonsmoking peers on film to impart information about three major social influences (family, peer, and media) and focused on immediate rather than long-term consequences of smoking. A pilot study of the program was implemented for four consecutive days to 750 seventh-grade students. The validity of self-reports of smoking behavior was improved by means of physiological monitoring. Students were shown a film indicating that their smoking could be detected from their saliva (nicotine analysis). While most samples were not actually analyzed, the expectation that they might be (known as the bogus pipeline technique, see Jones & Sigall, 1971) leads students to be more honest in their self-reports of smoking behavior (Evans, Hansen, & Mittlemark, 1977; Luepker, Pechacek, Murray, Johnson, Hurd, & Jacobs, 1981). Results of the pilot test indicated that, ten weeks after pretest, the proportion of nonsmokers in the combined experimental groups who previously had reported smoking at least one cigarette in the past month was approximately half that of the control group. However, these results are inconclusive in that results were just as large for a saliva-monitoring-only control group.

Research at both Stanford and Harvard (McAlister et al., 1979, 1980) and at Minnesota (Hurd et al., 1980; Murray, Johnson, Luepker, Pechacek, & Jacobs, 1980) expanded upon the basic model of inoculation with a persuasive communication. McAlister et al. (1979, 1980) developed a program, Counselling Leadership Against Smoking (project CLASP), which had the same features as that of Evans et al. (1978), with three important theory-based innovations. First, older student peer leaders (Hartup & Louge, 1975) were used to implement the program. Second, a session was introduced to increase social commitment not to smoke (derived from attribu-

tion theory, see Jones, Kanouse, Kelley, Nisbett, Valins, & Weiner, 1972).
Third, behavioral learning techniques, in the form of role-playing where
students act out situations requiring resistance to social pressure (derived
from social learning theory, see Bandura, 1977; Rotter, 1966), were introduced. The treatment consisted of three sessions on consecutive days, with
four booster sessions spaced over the remainder of the grade seven school
year. Results at nine months after pretest were impressive, with 5.6
percent of the experimental group reporting smoking during the previous
week, versus 9.9 percent in the control group.

The Robbinsdale Anti-Smoking Project (RASP) (Hurd, Johnson, &
Luepker, 1978; Hurd et al., 1980; Murray, Johnson, Luepker, Pechacek,
Jacobs, & Hurd, 1978) incorporates features of both the Evans et al.
program (1978) and CLASP, plus an additional innovative feature. Like
Evans' program, it does not use peer leaders to implement the program,
but uses peers in videotapes. As in CLASP, a public commitment component was added. This public commitment component used recognized
peer leaders (i.e., acquaintances) in the videotapes, which were intended
to increase source credibility and message salience. Classes were assigned
to one of five groups: (1) control; (2) intensive measurement only; (3) social
pressure curriculum and intensive measurement; (4) public commitment
plus social pressures curriculum and intensive measurement; and (5) per-
sonalization plus commitment, social pressure curriculum, and intensive
measurement. The results were encouraging. In the four experimental
groups combined, prevalence of regular smoking (at least once or twice a
month) had not increased at the rate that would have been expected had
there been no program by the end of the school year (nine months after
pretest). Smoking prevalence increased during the school year from 9.5
percent to 21.1 percent in group 2 and from 4.9 percent to 5.6 percent in
both group 4 and group 5. Saliva thiocyanate analyses were consistent with
self-report data (Luepker et al., 1981).

The Prevention of Cigarette Smoking in Children project (PCSC) (Murray et al., 1980) compared (1) a peer-led social-consequences program with
videotapes (similar to RASP), (2) a peer-led social-consequences program
without videotapes, and (3) an adult-led long-term health-consequences
program. At the end of the school year (nine months after pretest), the
peer-led social-consequences program without videotape (group 2) was
found the most effective in preventing onset of *regular smoking*. The
number of transitions from experimental to regular smoking was 60 percent
of that expected, as established by an external control group. With regard
to preventing *onset of experimentation*, however, the adult-led health-
consequences program (group 3) was the most effective (46 percent of
expected transitions) and the peer-led social-consequences program with
videotape (group 1) was least effective (76 percent of expected transitions).

Concurrently with work at Stanford, Harvard, and Minnesota, work on the Life Skills Training Program (LST) was begun at the American Health Foundation and continued at Cornell University Medical College (Botvin & Eng, 1980, 1982; Botvin et al., 1980; Botvin, Resnick, & Baker, 1981). LST attempted to address major psychological and social factors promoting the onset of smoking. The program aimed to teach students, in ten weekly sessions, the necessary skills to resist direct social pressures to smoke. It also tried to decrease students' susceptibility to indirect social pressures to smoke, by helping them develop greater autonomy, self-esteem, and self-confidence; and it attempted to provide students with a means of coping with anxiety induced by social situations. Results of this program, when implemented by allied health professionals, showed significantly fewer new smokers in the experimental school than in the control school during the last four weeks of training, at three-month posttest (4 percent vs. 16 percent), and at six-month follow-up (6 percent vs. 18 percent). A second study (Botvin & Eng, 1982), which utilized older leaders to conduct the program, indicated that, three months after pretest, significantly fewer of the students in the experimental group began smoking than in the control group (8 percent onset by previous nonsmokers in the experimental group versus 19 percent onset in control group).

The long-term effects of interventions on smoking have been investigated by several researchers. A three-year longitudinal study of Evans' program was undertaken in 13 schools to determine whether this program would deter smoking over the long term (Evans, Rozelle, Maxwell, Raines, Dill, Guthrie, Henderson, & Hill, 1981). Results showed that the full-treatment group had the highest percentage (6.8 percent) of frequent smokers (two or more cigarettes a day) at the end of the seventh grade (the first year of the intervention), as compared to a repeatedly tested control group (5.7 percent). By the end of eighth grade (the second year of intervention), however, the full-treatment group had the lowest percentage of frequent smokers (5.5 percent versus 11 percent), an effect that was maintained at the end of ninth grade (9.5 percent versus 14.2 percent). A similar pattern of results was obtained for intentions to smoke. Evans et al. (1980) advise caution in interpreting these results, due to the quasi-experimental nature of the study and the mode of analysis employed, which was successive cross-sectional rather than longitudinal. They have called for replication of these results to increase confidence in them.

Projects CLASP, RASP, and LST have provided some of the needed replication. Project CLASP reported data 21 months after pretest (McAlister et al., 1980), indicating that the effect of the program was maintained, with a 3.2 percent rate of onset of regular smoking in the experimental group versus an 8.4 percent onset rate in the control group. The RASP program reported follow-up data one year after pretest (Johnson, Luepker, Pechacek, Jacobs, & Hurd, 1979). Treatment effects were maintained, and the full-treatment experimental school was not taking up smoking at the rate that would have been expected had there been no program. This was indicated by the finding that, of those individuals who initially categorized themselves as either nonsmokers or as only experimenters, considerably more individuals from the measurement-only school categorized them-selves as regular smokers one year after pretest. Since this follow-up visit was unannounced, results cannot be explained by the fact that the program team's presence during the year simply postponed experimentation until they were gone. Long-term follow-ups of the LST program (Botvin & Eng, 1982; Botvin et al., 1981) have shown similarly maintained reductions in the onset of regular smoking, with approximately half as many of the nonsmokers in the program group as in the control group smoking at least weekly one year after the program. All research programs plan to continue monitoring for long-term effects.

A number of methodological concerns reduce the apparent impressive-ness of the results reported so far. Before accepting the consistency of results as evidence for the efficacy of social psychological smoking-prevention programs (Fisher, 1980), we need to consider their methodolo-gical strengths and weaknesses.

All of the reviewed studies were strong in at least three ways: (1) they all had both pretests and posttests, thus allowing for an assessment of changes over time; (2) they all included control groups, thus allowing for a compari-son of groups receiving the program with groups not receiving it; and (3) they all attempted to validate self-reports of smoking behavior by collecting physiological indicators, thus reducing the bias of self-reports by the use of the bogus-pipeline technique (Jones & Sigall, 1971).

The evaluation of preventive health behavior programs is a complex task, however (Flay & Best, 1982; Flay & Cook, 1981), and all of the reviewed studies have several methodological problems leaving the possibility that the observed effects could have been due to causes other than the smoking-prevention program. The first has to do with the small number of units, usually whole schools, assigned to each condition of an experimental design. Most studies had only one school per condition, and even these were not assigned randomly. In these studies, condition was confounded with school, so that any observed posttest differences could be due to characteristics of the school environment rather than the program. This criticism reduces the value of otherwise impressive results from the CLASP, RASP, and LST programs and, to a lesser extent, the PCSC program (where two schools were assigned randomly to each condition).

Future studies need to assign randomly many more schools, at least ten to each condition, before we can be confident that the observed effects are due to tested programs rather than characteristics of schools.

A second and related methodological problem concerns sample sizes. Most of the reviewed studies had a very small number of children in each condition. For example, having only zero to three children from any one grade level start smoking monthly in the treatment group while five or six did so in the control group (Botvin et al., 1980) cannot lead to any confidence that the finding is robust. This criticism also applies to the other studies reviewed. The low expected rates of smoking onset during the course of any one study means that larger sample sizes are imperative.

Another related issue concerns the appropriate unit of analysis. When schools are assigned randomly to conditions, and when the program is delivered to intact classes, the school is the most appropriate unit of statistical analysis for some purposes, while the classroom is most appropriate for others. It is not entirely appropriate to use individuals as the unit of analysis, except for those questions that concern the differential effects of different levels of treatment (e.g., attention to the program or performance of tasks within it).

A fourth methodological problem concerns the appropriateness of control groups. Most of the studies reviewed used essentially the same type of control group, a monitoring-only control. This control group does provide adequate protection against the possible effects of repeated monitoring. Evans et al. (1978) found that monitoring had as much effect as treatment, while Hurd et al. (1980) found that a testing-only group was no better than a self-report control group. We anticipate that testing will not be a serious problem unless the treatment being tested is a weak one; nevertheless, we probably should continue in future situations to isolate the effects of testing. Control groups that isolate the effects of testing, however, do not protect against Hawthorne effects. It is conceivable that some of the positive results reported to date have been due to the presence of outsiders in the schools treating students in a special way rather than to the content of the program.

Too few assessments of the effect of treatment beyond the end of the treatment year have been reported yet. It is important to determine whether or not the effects of preventive programs are maintained over time. It is possible that the long-term effects are greater as the smoking initiation rates increase in the control group. This may be particularly true of programs delivered early in the onset curve (grade six or seven). The smoking onset curve suggests that a smoking-prevention program is given most appropriately at grade six or seven, or even earlier, rather than grade ten, as some programs have done. By grade ten, most adolescents who are going to smoke already are smoking experimentally or regularly. This would suggest that programs at higher grades need to be addressed, in part, to getting regular smokers to quit (cf. Perry & Danaher, 1978; Perry, Telch, Killen, & Maccoby, 1980). An appropriately designed program for tenth graders also might prevent transitions from regular but infrequent (weekly) to heavy (pack-a-day) smoking (Johnson, personal communication, 1981).

The possible problem of attrition has hardly been addressed at all in reports of previous smoking-prevention research. This is due partly to the lack of completed long-term follow-ups; however, attrition can be a problem even over as short a period as one year. In Los Angeles, for example, we expect an attrition rate of close to 25 percent for any one year. In Waterloo, on the other hand, attrition over any 12-month period was 2.5 percent, only one-tenth as great. Future investigators are encouraged to provide information on attrition. Such information is particularly important when there is some chance that any attrition might be treatment related. It is likely that smokers, who also are more likely than nonsmokers to be doing poorly in school and have a low self-image of themselves, will leave school during treatment or be absent on testing occasions. The effects of such selective attrition on estimates of program effects need to be examined.

Finally, as programs are found to be effective, we need to try to find out why. One way of answering this question is to test alternatives, as Hurd et al. (1980) have done. This approach leads to very large studies, however, and results are not always very clear (Johnson, in press). Rather than trying to isolate program components, maybe we should follow educational researchers and test whole curricula (Schlegel et al., 1980). A combination of many elements is likely to be most effective, and it becomes unwieldy to attempt to separate out crucial components for testing. An alternative way of ascertaining what is most and least effective is a form of process evaluation. Each component of a program is designed to produce a particular effect, and it is the combination of all those effects that should prevent smoking. Evaluations should include measures of as many of these immediate and mediating effects as possible, in addition to measuring the final behavioral outcomes.

This review has shown that all previous evaluations of smoking-prevention programs have been limited in some respects; nevertheless, taken together, they represent promising support for the use of social inoculation, peer leaders, and coping-skills development techniques in smoking prevention. Our study at the University of Waterloo, to be reported on next, attempted to overcome most of the previously mentioned methodological problems; therefore, it provides the strongest test to date of the efficacy of the social psychological approach to smoking prevention.

The Waterloo Study

The University of Waterloo Study was based on (1) the correlates of smoking by youth reviewed earlier in this paper, (2) early reports of results from the social psychological programs reviewed previously in this chapter, (3) the methodological concerns also just discussed, and (4) a new model of the attitude and behavior change process. Before describing the program and its results, we first will describe its theoretical basis.

An Integrative Model of Attitude and Behavior Change. The complexity of the newer smoking-prevention programs suggests a need for a comprehensive model that would help in the design of better programs and in the identification of mediating variables to be assessed during evaluation

Figure 6.4   Integrative Model of Health Attitude and Behavior Change.

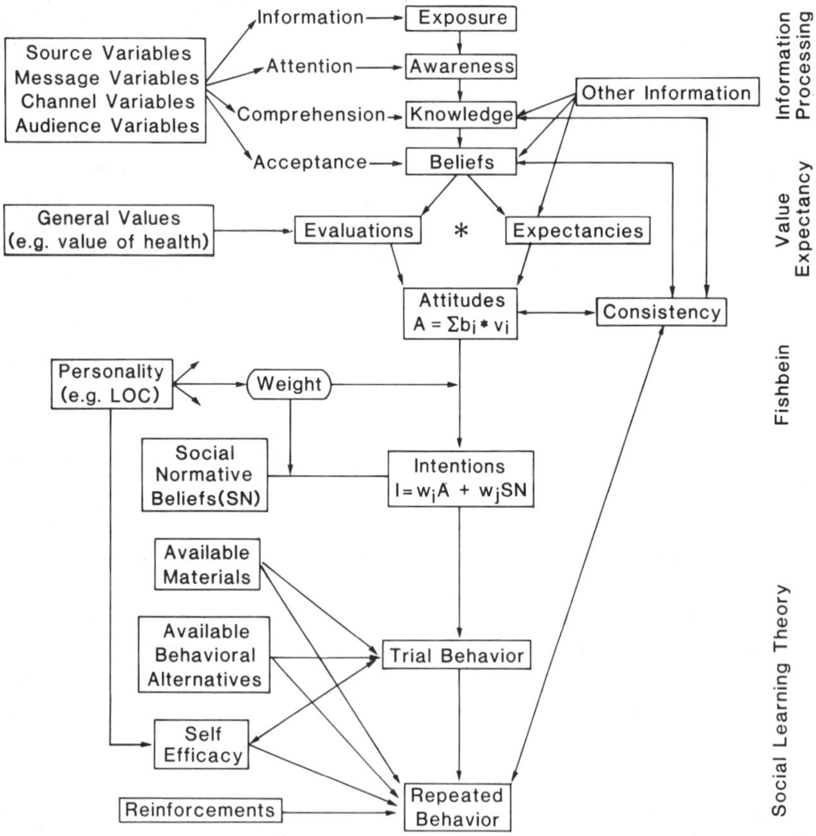

(McAlister, 1981; Perry, in press). The following model of the communication process (Figure 6.4), developed by one of us (Flay, 1979, 1981), is an integration of much social psychological research and theory.

First, much is known about how, or the conditions under which, information leads to changes in knowledge and beliefs. The information-processing model developed at Yale (Hovland, Lumsdaine, & Sheffield, 1949; Hovland, Janis, & Kelly, 1953) and elaborated upon by McGuire (1969, 1972, 1978) provides the best description of this process. Information provided by a credible and familiar source, in an appropriate form (message variables), via appropriate channels, if attended to and comprehended, will lead to changes in knowledge, and if accepted will lead to desired changes in beliefs. For children, the most effective strategies would include providing information about immediate consequences, rather than long-term ones, presented by "peer leaders" with appropriate repetition by other sources, along with the use of active generation of information and arguments by the audience.

An obvious shortcoming of the information-processing model is that it assumes that changes in knowledge and beliefs will lead automatically to changes in attitudes and behavior. Changes in knowledge and beliefs will not necessarily lead to changes in attitudes unless values also are considered. The best known explanation of this step is provided by the value-expectancy formulations of Fishbein (1967; Fishbein & Ajzen, 1974, 1975), the health-belief model (Hochbaum, 1958; Maiman & Becker, 1974; Rosenstock, 1974), Rogers' model (1975) for the effects of fear communications, and others (see reviews by Beck & Frankel, 1981; Feather, 1982; Lutz, 1981; Maiman & Becker, 1974). The form of these models is shown at the second level in Figure 6.4. The value-expectancy formulations suggest that in order to change children's attitudes we should focus on (1) the consequences to which they feel vulnerable or susceptible and which they perceive as noxious or severe and (2) the likelihood and value of the positive consequences of not smoking. Specific and immediate, rather than general and long-term, consequences should be most salient in these respects. Just as predicted by the information-processing model, active and self-generated strategies are likely to be more effective than passive acquisition. Thus, group discussion and the decision-balance-sheet technique of Janis & Mann (1977) might be good ways of ensuring the salience of expectancies and their corresponding values.

Although most discussions of value-expectancy theories focus on predicting intentions or behavior, these theories really are applied appropriately only to predicting attitudes toward a behavior. In order for intentions to be predicted, we also must consider social-normative beliefs (i.e., social norms, influences, or pressures) regarding that behavior. Thus, Fishbein's model for predicting intentions from attitudes and social-normative beliefs provides the next link in the integrative model (see the third level of Figure 6.4). With regard to children and smoking behavior, we believe that normative beliefs (e.g., family or peer influences) are more important determinants of behavior at younger ages, while attitudes become more important in late adolescence.

Personality factors are probably most important at this point in the model, although their effects may be rather pervasive (hence the multiple arrows in Figure 6.4). It is known that people who are more internally controlled place greater weight on their own attitudes in determining their attitudes toward a behavior than on the more externally derived normative beliefs (Saltzer, 1978). It is also known that older adolescents are more likely to be internally controlled than are younger children (Lefcourt, 1972; Parcel & Meyer, 1978). Thus, we would expect that, as adolescents become older, their attitudes toward smoking will become more important determinants of their intentions and, we hope, of their behavior, than social pressures. Alternatively, training youngsters to resist social pressures might make them more internally controlled.

Changing behavioral intentions will not necessarily lead to attempting the corresponding behavior unless individuals either (1) feel that they possess or can acquire control over the requisite new behavior (self-efficacy in Figure 6.4); and/or (2) possess alternative behavioral skills for coping with pressures that will enable them to act in the positive, new way. Recent behavioral formulations emphasize the development of specific coping skills (Bandura, 1977). For the prevention of smoking onset, the relevant skills include those necessary to resist successfully the social pressures that are such important determinants of smoking onset.

Once a behavior is tried, there is no guarantee that it will be repeated or maintained. Maintenance of a behavior requires that it be practiced and reinforced. Thus, a smoking-prevention program needs to include opportunities to practice the new behavioral skills being taught, as well as reinforcement for appropriate behavior. Approaches derived from attribution theory, where children who are told that they are good at something become good at it (Miller, Brickman, & Bolan, 1975), also might be useful at this point.

Finally, the many consistency theories in social psychology (Abelson, Aronson, McGuire, Newcomb, Rosenberg, & Tannebaum, 1968) suggest that changes anywhere in the model shown in Figure 6.4 would help create changes in other areas because of the drive toward consistency. Thus, change need not always occur in the order described, but could occur in almost any order. We suspect that consistency might not be as important for children as for adolescents. Programs probably can be more effective if they draw attention to each of a person's beliefs, attitudes, values, and behaviors, and so indirectly exert pressure toward consistency.

To summarize, the integrative model shown in Figure 6.4 suggests that information, if it is attended to, comprehended and accepted, may lead to changes in beliefs; but beliefs will not necessarily lead to changes in attitudes, unless values and expectancies are considered; attitudes will not necessarily lead to changes in intentions unless social influences are considered; and intentions will not necessarily lead to behavioral responses unless the individual has the necessary control and coping skills. This model makes clear why earlier smoking-education programs tended to fail. They focused their intervention efforts toward the top of the model and did not give enough attention to elements closer to behavior. Even most value-clarification programs are focused near the top of the model. Programs that include decision-making skills may influence intentions but will not change behavior directly. Those programs providing both coping skills and image-building (which is likely to influence self-efficacy and social reinforcement contingencies), together with peer-group strategies (working on social-normative beliefs) and affective skills training, are likely to be most effective, according to this model. The reported evaluations of smoking-education and -prevention programs and of more general drug education programs seem to be consistent with such an expectation.

Program Content.   The content of the University of Waterloo Smoking Prevention Program was designed to be consistent with the known correlates (and suspected causes) of smoking and the model of attitude and behavior change just described. The program has three major components, delivered in six one-hour weekly sessions during grade six.

1.   The first component, and the first two sessions, focus on providing information about the consequences of smoking and the reasons for smoking. While the focus is on information, the activities are designed to start the development of future attitude and behavior changes and the acquisition of social skills. The information is elicited from the children rather than provided for them. This approach has three major advantages. First, it forces the children to search through their belief systems. This is important in that many children believe categorically that smoking is bad, but have few supportive beliefs. Elicitation of beliefs therefore helps them to discover that they have little information upon which to base their beliefs, and this in turn should encourage them to begin to search their environment for more information. Searching for information then is encouraged explicitly and reinforced throughout the remainder of the program. A second advantage of eliciting information is that the information provided will be more salient than if it came from a teacher. Finally, information gathered collectively from a classroom usually provides a comprehensive coverage of the beliefs of the immediate peer group. The information discussed also is repeated via multiple modes, such as video tapes, poster making, role

playing, and class discussion, to increase the probability of attention, comprehension, and rentention.

2.   The second component of the program focuses on the social influences (family, peer, media, and other) that encourage smoking, and develops skills to resist such pressures. Again, information is elicited as much as possible from the children, and repetition is achieved by the use of multiple modalities. In the fourth session, specific social-coping skills are taught, role played, and practiced. Practice includes videotaped feedback of performance and provisions for opportunities to improve skills.

3.   This final component of the program is concerned with decision making and public commitment. Children are asked to integrate the information learned in all previous sessions and to make a decision about starting to smoke. They are provided with a tool for decision making, the decisional balance sheet of Janis & Mann (1977), for which they list (1) harms to myself if I smoke, (2) harms to others if I smoke, (3) benefits to myself if I smoke, (4) benefits to others if I smoke, (5) who will disapprove if I smoke, and (6) who will approve if I smoke. Based on these lists, each child makes a decision about future smoking and indicates the main reason for that decision. Finally, in the public commitment procedure, they announce their decisions, along with their main reasons for them, to their classmates. These public announcements are videotaped, purportedly to be shown to future grade six children.

This program, known as the core program, is delivered during the first two months of grade six. Two additional sessions, called maintenance sessions, are given later in grade six. These are designed to keep the issues, skills, and decisions salient. Finally, two additional booster sessions are provided during grades seven and eight. These are thought to be important, because the students will be exposed to increasing peer pressure at this age.

Program Evaluation.   The evaluation of the University of Waterloo Program was designed to overcome as many of the previously discussed methodological problems as possible. The protocol called for 24 schools to be assigned randomly to treatment and control conditions.

In the Waterloo County Separate School Board, 17 schools that met the criteria volunteered to participate. The criteria were (1) that the students stay in the same school from grade six to grade eight, rather than changing at grade seven, (2) that the schools be willing to be assigned randomly to experimental or control conditions, (3) that all grade six students in a selected school participate in the study, and (4) that the schools make a commitment to participate in all intervention and evaluation procedures for the 32 months of the study. Twelve of the 17 volunteer schools were matched on urban/rural location (one rural and five urban pairs) and socioeconomic status (SES) as judged by the superintendent of schools; the schools then were assigned randomly to condition.

In the Oxford County Board of Education, all ten of the schools that were asked to participate were rural (and located outside of the tobacco growing areas within the county). Assignment again was made after matching on SES. Randomization was not completely successful in that some principals had their schools assigned to the treatment condition because it was known they would not cooperate if they were not receiving the program. Subsequent analyses do not suggest that any biases were caused by this procedure.

All grade six classes in each of the schools participated in the study. In most cases there was only one grade six class per school. Both treatment and control schools were, or will be, measured at a pretest, at an immediate posttest, and at follow-ups at the end of grade six and at the beginning and end of grades seven and eight. Thus, the study encompasses a three-year period. At the time of this writing, subjects are at the end of grade seven. Most of the results to be reported here are confined to data collected prior to and at the beginning of grade seven. At the time of writing, data from the end of grade seven had only just become available and had not yet been analyzed in any detail. The design does not control for Hawthorne effects; a subsequent study planned for 1982 is designed to do this.

A questionnaire was designed to assess most of the components of the integrative model shown in Figure 6.4. The questionnaire also included demographic information and assesses the smoking habits of parents, siblings, peers, and teachers. Smoking is measured by self-report; to increase the validity of self-report, samples of saliva are collected and analyzed for thiocyanate.

The data appear to be of high quality. Ninety-four percent of children in the total sample received parental consent, providing a study sample of 697 children in 22 schools. Attrition over one year due to children changing classes or schools was only 2.5 percent, compared to ten or more in most studies. Absenteeism was close to 5 percent (also typically ten percent or more in other studies) for any one session, including testing sessions. There was a high level of satisfaction with the program. At the end of the core program, program components were rated on five-point scales by the children in terms of liking, length, difficulty, learning, and interest. Eighty-four percent of them liked the program; 72 percent thought it was the right length; 81 percent thought it was just the right level of difficulty; 96 percent felt they had learned something from it; and 74 percent found it interesting. The regular classroom teachers, who observed the program as it was delivered by specially trained health education specialists, felt that all program components were effective teaching methods.

Pretest Data.   Experimental and control groups did not differ at pretest with respect to (1) smoking; (2) gender; (3) prevalence of parental, sibling, or peer smoking; (4) beliefs; (5) attitudes; (6) social-normative beliefs; (7) intentions with respect to smoking; or (8) locus of control. They did differ with respect to knowledge, with the control group being more knowledgeable, responding correctly to 4.89 of nine items, as compared to 4.76 items for the experimentals [$\chi^2(6) = 79.48, p < .0001$]. The difference is in the opposite direction from the experimental hypothesis for program effects, and this makes the estimate of program effects more conservative than it otherwise might be. The two groups also were significantly different in age, with the control group being older (11.11 years) than the experimental group (10.91 years) [$\chi^2(3) = 17.7, p < .0005$]. Because age typically correlates positively with prevalence of smoking, this difference could be confounded with the program effects and will need to be adjusted out. However, the few differences found between treatment and control groups were minimal and did not seriously affect the interpretability of the overall results.

The following categories were used to score smoking behavior for each subjects:

1. *Never-smokers:* subjects who reported having never smoked, not even one puff of a cigarette
2. *Quitters:* subjects who had smoked, even if only once, but had quit
3. *Experimenters:* subjects who had not quit, but smoked less than once a week
4. *Regular smokers:* subjects who reported smoking at least once a week

At pretest, 42 percent of the total sample were never-smokers, another 42 percent were quitters (about half had tried only one cigarette or less), 12 percent were experimenters, and only 4 percent were regular smokers. These figures closely replicated those of Brown et al. (1978) on a similar sample. Males showed higher rates of regular and experimental smoking at pretest (18 percent) than did females (12 percent), which also replicated the findings of Brown et al. (1978). Also as expected, increased age was associated with increased rates of onset, as shown in Table 6.1.

The data clearly and strongly replicated the usual relationships between social influences and smoking. Table 6.2 shows the pretest relationship between parental smoking and the subjects' smoking onset status. The prevalence of smoking increased linearly as the number of smoking parents increased, [$\chi^2(2) = 21.0, p < .0^001$]. Despite the fact that more boys than girls were smoking, it appeared that the parental influence was greater on same-gender offspring, [$\chi^2(2) = 3.03, p < .04$]. If the father smoked, 75 percent of the sons had tried smoking by grade six, while only 53 percent of the daughters had. The trend was reversed if mother smoked,

Table 6.1
Smoking Category by Age at Pretest (number and percent)

Age	Never-Smokers	Quitters	Experimenters	Regular Smokers	
9	2	1	0	0	N = 3
	66.67*	33.33	0.00	0.00	
10	60	39	9	2	
	54.55	35.45	8.18	1.82	N = 110
11	193	186	53	12	
	43.47	41.89	11.94	2.70	N = 444
12	18	44	11	8	
	22.22	54.32	13.58	9.98	N = 81
13	0	9	4	2	
	0.00	60.00	26.67	13.33	N = 15

*Row percent

Table 6.2
Behavioral Group by Parental Smoking (pretest)

Parental Smoking	Smoking Category				
	Never-Smokers	Quitters	Experimenters	Regular Smokers	
Neither	135	99	19	6	
parent	49.45*	35.48	24.67	25.00	N = 259
smokes	52.12**	38.22	7.33	2.31	
Father	54	63	21	10	
only	19.78	22.58	27.27	41.66	N = 148
smokes	36.48	42.56	14.18	6.75	
Mother	40	47	10	3	
only	14.65	16.84	12.98	12.50	N = 100
smokes	40.00	47.00	10.00	3.00	
Both	44	70	27	5	
parents	16.11	25.08	35.06	20.83	N = 146
smoke	30.13	47.94	18.49	3.42	

*Column percent
**Row percent

with 64 percent of the daughters having tried while only 56 percent of the sons had.

If a brother or sister smoked, only 20 percent of the sample had never smoked and 32 percent currently were smoking. In contrast, if there was no sibling smoking, 45 percent had never smoked and only 12 percent currently were smoking $[\chi^2(2) = 9.2, p < .01]$. This effect was confounded, of course, with the influence of parental smoking on sibling smoking.

Peer influence was correlated very highly with smoking behavior, as can be seen in Table 6.3. Eighty-six percent of the experimenters and all of the regular smokers had friends who smoked. In comparison, only 33 percent of the never-smokers reported having friends who smoked. Similar relationships were evident for the other smoking categories.

Results. At the immediate posttest, experimental and control groups differed in smoking behavior $[\chi^2(3) = 16.7, p < .0008]$. As can be seen in Figure 6.5, the difference appeared to be largely due to quitting on the part of students in the experimental group who already were smoking at pretest. In neither group was there yet a significant increase in smoking. By the end of grade six, any difference between groups had dissipated, and the two groups no longer differed significantly in smoking behavior. This program, however, was not designed to produce cessation. To the extent that it occurred, it was an unexpected, positive side-effect.

The intended effects of the program began to emerge by the beginning of grade seven, $[\chi^2(3) = 9.67, p < .02]$. As can be seen in Figure 6.6, the effects were due largely to an increased level of experimenting in the control group, which was not seen in the experimental group. It is important to note that the beginning of grade seven was the first point at which this program effect could be expected. Provision of the program at the grade six level was chosen deliberately because the available epidemiolo-

Table 6.3
Smoking Category by Friends' Smoking Behavior (number and percent)

Friends Smoke?	Smoking Category				
	Never-Smokers	Quitters	Experimenters	Regular Smokers	
None	183	114	10	0	
	67.03*	40.86	12.99	0.00	N = 307
Some	86	149	55	16	
	31.50	53.41	71.43	66.67	N = 306
Many	4	11	10	5	
	1.47	3.94	12.99	20.83	N = 30
All	0	3	1	3	
	0.00	1.08	1.30	12.50	N = 7
Don't Know	0	2	1	0	
	0.00	.72	1.30	0.00	N = 3

*Column percent

Figure 6.5 Categories of Smoking Behavior by Experimental Condition at Immediate Posttest.

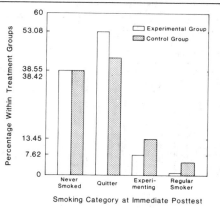

Smoking Category at Immediate Posttest

gical data (Brown et al., 1978; Johnston et al., 1977, 1979) suggested that smoking onset first becomes significant in grade seven, and we wanted to anticipate this increase with the preventive program. It was expected that this observed difference at the beginning of grade seven would increase considerably over time as the rate of smoking onset in the control group increased. Preliminary data from the end of grade seven (see Figure 6.6) confirm this expectation.

Table 6.4 shows that program effects by grade seven occurred in most behavioral categories. The program had no effect on the number of children remaining never-smokers. It increased the number of quitters, and these quitters came from all other categories; that is, even some prior nonsmokers, as well as experimenters and regular smokers, became quitters. As already shown, the program almost halved the number of children becoming experimenters by the beginning of grade seven. This effect also came from all other behavioral categories; that is, fewer nonsmokers, prior quitters, and regular smokers in the treatment group became experimenters by grade seven than in the control group. While the program does not appear to have reduced the number of children becoming regular smokers, the total number of regular smokers is really too small to afford us any firm conclusions.

Program effects are seen to be much larger in all behavioral categories when students who are at high risk of becoming smokers are examined. We defined high-risk students as those with two or more smoking parents, siblings, or friends. As noted earlier, high-risk students were much more likely than other students to have tried smoking already by the beginning of grade six. Table 6.5 shows that high-risk students also were very likely to

Figure 6.6   Percentage of Students Experimenting with Smoking at Pre-test and Four Posttests by Experimental Condition.

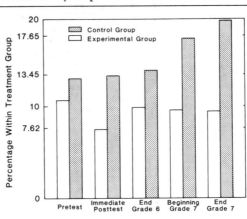

be influenced by the smoking-prevention program. Among those high-risk students who had never tried smoking by the beginning of grade six, none who received the program had done so by the beginning of grade seven, while 12 percent of those in the control group had done so. Among those who defined themselves as quitters at pretest, 23 percent of those in the control group had become experimenters one year later, as compared to only 14 percent in the treatment group. Sixty-one percent of those high-risk students in the treatment group who were experimenters in grade six had decided to quit by grade seven, versus only 36 percent in the control group. Although the N's are small, high-risk students in the treatment group who were regular smokers at pretest were much more likely than those in the control group to quit by grade seven.

The integrative model of attitude and behavior change suggests that long-term program impact, in terms of deterrence of smoking onset, might be mediated by changes in knowledge, beliefs, attitudes, intentions, and other variables, as they interact with individual differences. As noted earlier, the control group was significantly more knowledgeable at pretest. By the immediate posttest, however, the difference had been reversed, $[\chi^2(7) = 90.8, p < .0001]$, as the program resulted in marked knowledge acquisition by the experimental group ($\bar{X} = 5.76$). This difference was maintained through the end of grade six $[\bar{X} = 5.41, \chi^2(7) = 50.1, p < .0001]$ and the beginning of grade seven $[\bar{X} = 5.18, \chi^2(7) = 58.6, p < .0001]$, although with some decay.

Findings similar to those for knowledge have not been repeated yet with beliefs, attitudes, or intentions, largely because of marked ceiling effects.

Table 6.4

Transition Table (all Subjects): Percent within Each Smoking Category at Age 14 by Smoking Category at Pretest and Experimental Condition

Present Category	Condition*	Never	Quit	Experimenter	Regular	N(Row)	%(Col)
NEVER	T	76.5	20.5	1.5	1.5	136	42.4
	C	80.5	14	5	1	108	42.3
QUIT	T	0	83.5	11	6	139	43.3
	C	0	76	18	6	105	41.2
EXPERIMENTER	T	0	59.5	27	13.5	37	11.5
	C	0	37	50	13	30	11.8
REGULAR	T	0	22	33	44	9	2.8
	C	0	8	50	42	12	4.7
N (Col)	T	104	168	30	19	321	
	C	87	107	45	16	255	
% (Row)	T	32.3	52.3	9	5.9		
	C	34.1	41.9	17.6	6.2		

* T = Treatment (Program)
   C = Control

Table 6.5

Transition Table for High-Risk Subjects: Percent within Each Smoking Category at Age 14 by Smoking Category at Pretest and Experimental Conditions

PRETEST CATEGORY	CONDITIONS	CATEGORY AT T4				N
		NEVER	QUIT	EXPERIMENTER	REGULAR	
NEVER	T	74	26	0	0	23
	C	63	25	8	4	24
QUIT	T	0	76	14	10	59
	C	0	65	23	12	48
EXPERIMENTER	T	0	61	26	13	23
	C	0	36	52	12	25
REGULAR	T	0	29	29	43	7
	C	0	0	44	56	9

Figure 6.7   Mean Personalized Belief Score by Smoking Category at Pretest.

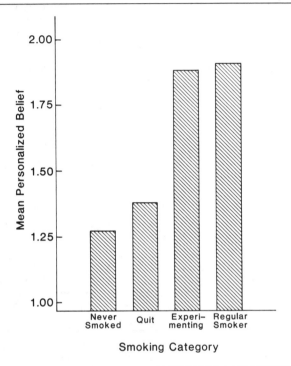

Young children have undifferentiated beliefs and attitudes toward smoking (they simply *think* it is bad), and this unitary evaluation was reflected in the various ratings. Cross-sectional data (Figure 6.7) showed a correlation between beliefs and experience with smoking. Only longitudinal data will determine whether beliefs or behavior change first, but it is possible that with increasing age and experience with smoking these beliefs, attitudes, and intentions are likely to become more differentiated, resulting in the program effects on them becoming apparent.

The program also caused some significant differences in a smoking-specific measure of locus of control. There were three subscales (Parcel & Meyer, 1978): internal or personal control, control by powerful others, and chance or fate. At immediate posttest, the experimental group was more internal than the control group on the personal control subscale [$\chi^2(7) = 21.4, p < .003$]. At the end of grade six, the experimental group was more internal on the chance subscale [$\chi^2(4) = 13.28, p < .01$]. The effects were less consistent than for knowledge, but were in the expected direction.

Discussion.   The low attrition rates, high cooperation of school personnel and students, and the ratings of interest in the program suggest that the program was delivered well to all recipients and that the evaluative data were of high quality. Pretest differences between treatment and control groups were minimal, showing that the assignment to conditions, although not entirely random, was successful. The short-term program effects on smoking behavior were in the expected direction and relatively consistent. It is encouraging that these effects were seen as early as the beginning of grade seven. The numbers of students smoking and the differences between treatment and control are still small and the findings are preliminary; however, with continuing follow-up through the end of grade eight, the study should be able to show significant effects and also demonstrate whether or not short-term effects are maintained. As more data from later time periods become available, it will be important to adjust for the effects of predictors of smoking stage in estimating program effects. Of further interest will be the relationships between changes in the various mediating and process variables of the models of Figures 6.3 and 6.4.

Implications for Future Program Development and Research

Traditional educational approaches to smoking prevention have been unsuccessful. More recent social psychologically derived programs have been more successful, but there is still much we do not know about how well, why, and for whom they work. In this section we discuss ways in which the success of future smoking-prevention programs and the research on them might be improved.

While the social psychologically derived programs are a distinct improvement over traditional educational approaches, they still fail to address adequately some of the major antecedents of smoking. For example, adolescents' desires for maturity, autonomy, or sexual sophistication, often attributed to the smoker, are not addressed adequately. There may be some acknowledgment of the "tough" and "cool" image of a smoker, but little attempt has been made to deal directly with this factor. Thus, these programs may succeed with children who might try smoking as a result of peer pressure, but they may be less effective with those who want to experiment with taking on the air of rebelliousness and sexual sophistication that they associate with being a smoker (Leventhal & Cleary, 1980).

Past programs have been designed to be suitable for the "average" adolescent. Thus, sixth- or seventh-grade children were provided with the program because the major rise in the onset curve occurs during junior high school. However, our own data showed that many of the high-risk adolescents already were smoking by grade six; that is, 35 percent of those children with two smoking parents already were experimenting and 20 percent already were regular smokers, compared with only 12 percent and 4 percent, respectively, for the total sample. Similarly, 26 percent of individuals with any friends who smoked already were experimenters or regular smokers. Two important implications follow from these figures. First, smoking-prevention programs may have to be provided even earlier than grade six in order to catch high-risk individuals. Second, programs may need to address more adequately the issue of how to counteract the strong modeling influence of smoking parents, siblings, and friends. The success of our program on high-risk subjects was gratifying.

Most of the programs reviewed were confined to a small number of sessions, usually during one grade. This seems unwise for two reasons. First, we know that most changes in the cognitive and affective domains do not persist over time (Cook & Flay, 1978). Thus, the more time that passes before knowledge or skills are used, the more likely they are to decline. This cannot be rectified by providing the program later, for the reasons given previously. Therefore, there is a need for providing longer and more cumulative programs, ones that review information and reinforce skills learned in earlier sessions. One way of doing this is to provide maintenance and booster sessions throughout the later grades, as is being done at the University of Waterloo. While this was a step forward, we now do not believe it to be sufficient. Rather, the developmental nature of the process of becoming a smoker suggests that preventive efforts should be spread throughout the developmental sequence (i.e., for five to ten years).

The neglect of the developmental nature of the process of becoming a smoker might be a major reason for the limited success of smoking-prevention programs to date. The developmental nature of the process has several implications for programming. First, it suggests that different procedures might be appropriate for different stages. It probably requires a different type of program content to prevent individuals ever trying their first cigarette than it does to prevent people from experimenting further or becoming regular smokers. Our model suggests, for example, that social influences may not be as important for the transition from experimental smoking to regular smoking as they are for the onset of experimental smoking. Second, different procedures might be appropriate for different age groups (regardless of their stages of smoking). It is necessary to draw on the knowledge of developmental psychologists to help understand how a child's beliefs, attitudes, and responses to social influences develop over time; how they affect smoking behavior; and how changes in them might best be brought about.

Yet another reason for the limited success of smoking-prevention programs is the almost total neglect of the broader social environment. All the school-based programs reviewed, and most of the other types not reviewed (cf. Leventhal & Cleary, 1981), were directed at the individual. But individuals exist in a social environment that has pervasive influences. A program that actively involves families, friends, schools, the medical profession, media events, and community action is more likely to be effective than a program that focuses exclusively on children in the classroom. (See Flay, Hansen, Johnson, Alvarez, Sobal, Simmons, Kaufman, & Ulene, 1982 for an example of the application of this suggestion in the area of smoking-prevention programming.)

Some of these suggestions on how smoking programs might be improved rely on basic knowledge and theory that either does not exist yet or is incomplete. For example, developing a long-term, cumulative program that takes into account the stages involved in becoming a smoker requires a good theory of that process. While the model presented in Figure 6.3 might be a good start, knowledge and theory in which we can have much more confidence are needed. Development of this knowledge base requires interdisciplinary studies of a prospective and longitudinal nature. Some of these studies need to be large population surveys, and some need to be more ecological in nature, involving the intensive observation of children as they develop. The model of Figure 6.3 and others like it should be considered only as starting points.

Before planning a program that takes into account the developmental stage of students, a detailed understanding is needed of the development over time of children's beliefs, attitudes, and responses to social influences, as well as the structural relationships among these. Of even greater importance is the need to know how experience with smokers and/or smoking affect this development, and how changes in this experience might be brought about in order to change how it affects the child's own smoking behavior. Another area where good basic understanding is lacking concerns children's understanding or perceptions of group, community, and society values and norms and how these perceptions affect their desire to try cigarettes, experiment with them, or become regular smokers. Such understanding is necessary before highly successful programs involving many sections of society can be developed.

Because of the deficiencies of basic knowledge and the resulting lack of good theory, past smoking-prevention programs have not been grounded adequately in comprehensive theory. If they had been, they might not have neglected the five issues we have just discussed. While the social psychologically based programs are much more sophisticated in their use of theory than earlier programs, even they are rather limited. They focus on the social influences in the development of smoking, often to the neglect of

Figure 6.8 Integrating a Model of the Development of Smoking Behavior and a Model of the Attitude and Behavior Change Process.

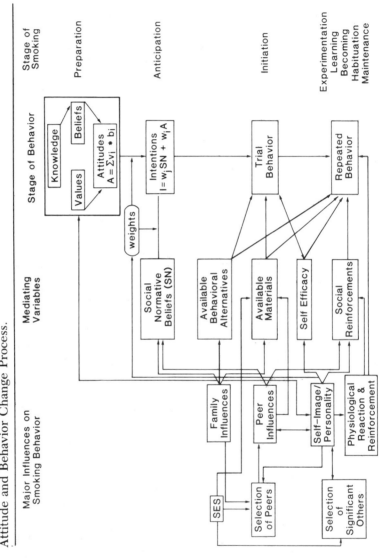

170

other equally important influences. Even our own use of an integrative model of the attitude and behavior change process is not sufficient in that it focuses on the communication process rather than the process of becoming a smoker. Both foci are necessary for effective program development and evaluation. An attempt at considering both foci is shown in Figure 6.8, an integration of Figures 6.3 and 6.4. This model demonstrates how basic theoretical knowledge from psychology supports the idea that the importance of different influencing variables changes as an individual develops.

Knowledge and theory both would be improved if evaluations of smoking prevention programs incorporated much more process evaluation. There are several different kinds of process evaluation mentioned in the literature, all of which could contribute to better theory. One type, alternatively known as implementation assessment, involves assessing exactly what was delivered to who, by whom, and under what conditions. Reports of past smoking-prevention program evaluations give us very little idea of exactly what the program was or how it was delivered. Without such information a science of intervention can never be developed because it is impossible for true replication to occur.

A second type of process evaluation is concerned with the "strength" of a program (Sechrest, West, Phillips, Redner, & Yeaton, 1979). Somewhat analogous to "manipulation checks" in social psychology, this involves an assessment of how well each component of a program or lesson curriculum is meeting its objectives. Each session of a smoking-prevention program presumably is meant to change something, which then may lead to later behavior changes. Such changes in knowledge, beliefs, attitudes, perceptions of social norms, social and/or coping skills, and possibly even personality ought to be measured. To the extent that any one or more of them is not changed successfully by the program, behavior change is less likely to occur, or changes are less likely to be maintained.

A third type of process evaluation is concerned with moderator variables; that is, variables that will not be changed by the program but that nevertheless influence the target behavior. This type of process evaluation would require assessment of variables like SES, parental behavior and attitudes, friends' behavior and attitudes, society and community norms, and so on—all constructs presented in Figure 6.3 that are not expected to be changed by the program. The mediating influence of these variables on program effectiveness then can be examined. If this type of process evaluation had been done in the past, we already might have found, for example, whether or not it was a waste of time and resources to provide a program to sixth-grade children with parents who smoke. Perhaps high-risk groups need the program earlier, or even a different program.

In conclusion, concentrating on outcome evaluation to the exclusion of process evaluation is no longer a useful approach. The strong test provided

by the University of Waterloo Study confirms that social psychologically
derived smoking-prevention programs can be efficacious. They can have
effects that not only are statistically significant, but also are of great
practical importance, approximately halving the number of children who
experiment with cigarette smoking, at least in the short-term. The only
plausible alternative explanation of those effects that remains to be ruled
out by future studies is the Hawthorne effect. It is unlikely that the
Hawthorne effect can account for more than a minor portion of the large
effect obtained, so finding that attention is responsible for a part of the
effect probably would not be of serious practical concern. An important
area of unanswered questions concerns program dissemination. Will these
programs be as successful when implemented on a wide scale by regular
classroom teachers? Ongoing research by each of the major groups involved in smoking-prevention research is designed to explore this question. Experimental evaluations still are required for assessments of the
Hawthorne effect and approaches to program dissemination. In addition,
however, process evaluation now is necessary to help advance our knowledge and theory about how smoking behavior develops and how it might
best be altered. We should not let the demands for quick solutions distract
us from efforts, both in basic research and in process evaluation, to trace
the complex processes involved. Some guidelines for the directions the
basic research might take, as well as preliminary models to be tested and
modified, have been provided in this chapter.

References

Abelson, R. P., Aronson, E., McGuire, W. J., Newcomb, T. M., Rosenberg, M. J.,
    & Tannebaum, P. H. (eds.). *Theories of cognitive consistency: A source
    book*. Chicago: Rand McNally, 1968.
Allegrante, J. P., O'Rourke, T. W., & Tuncalp, S. A multivariate analysis of
    selected psychosocial variables in the development of subsequent youth
    smoking behavior. *Journal of Drug Education*, 1977, *1*, 237–248.
American Cancer Society. *A study of public school teachers' cigarette smoking
    attitudes and habits*. New York, N.Y.: American Cancer Society, 1976.
Baer, D. J. & Katkin, J. M. Imitation of smoking by sons and daughters who smoke
    and smoking behavior of parents. *Journal of Genetic Psychology*, 1971, *118*,
    293–296.
Bandura, A. *Social learning theory*. Englewood Cliffs, N.J.: Prentice-Hall, 1977.
Baric, L. Non-smokers, smokers, ex-smokers: Three separate problems for health
    education. *International Journal of Health Education*, 1979, *22*, 2–20.
Baric, L., & Fischer, C. Acquisition of the smoking habit. *Health Education
    Journal*, 1979, *38*, 71–76.
Beaglehole, R., Eyles, E., & Harding, W. A controlled smoking intervention

progamme in secondary schools. *New Zealand Medical Journal*, 1978, *87*, 278–280.

Beck, K. H., & Frankel, A. A conceptualization of threat communications and protective health behavior. *Social Psychology Quarterly*, 1981, *44*:3, 204–217.

Bentler, P. M. Multivariate analysis with latent variables: Causal modelling. *Annual Review of Psychology*, 1980, *31*, 419–456.

Bergin, J. I., & Wake, F. R. Report to the Department of National Health and Welfare on Canadian research on psycho-social aspects of cigarette smoking: 1960–1972. Ottawa, Canada: Canadian Department of National Health and Welfare, 1974.

Bernstein, D. A., & McAlister, A. The modification of smoking behavior: Progress and problems. *Addictive Behaviors*, 1976, *1*, 89–102.

Best, J. A., & Bloch, M. Compliance in the control of cigarette smoking. In R. B. Haynes, D. W. Taylor, & D. L. Sackett (eds.), *Compliance with therapeutic and preventive regimens*. Baltimore: Johns Hopkins University Press, 1979.

Bewley, B., & Bland, J. M. Smoking and respiratory symptoms in two groups of school children. *Preventive Medicine*, 1976, *5*, 63–69.

Bewley, B. R., Bland, J. M., & Harris, R. Factors associated with the starting of cigarette smoking by primary school children. *British Journal of Preventive and Social Medicine*, 1974, *28*, 37–44.

Bewley, B. R., Halil, T., & Snaith, A. H. Smoking in primary school children. Prevalence and associated respiratory symptoms. *British Journal of Preventive and Social Medicine*, 1973, *27*, 150–153.

Borland, B. L. Relative effects of low socio-economic status, parental smoking and poor scholastic performance on smoking among high school students. *Social Science and Medicine*, 1975, *9*, 27–30.

Botvin, G., & Eng, A. A comprehensive school-based smoking prevention program. *Journal of School Health*, 1980, 209–213.

Botvin, G., & Eng, A. The efficacy of a multicomponent approach to the prevention of cigarette smoking. *Preventive Medicine*, 1982, *11*, 199–211.

Botvin, G., Eng, A., & Williams C. Preventing the onset of smoking through life skills training. *Preventive Medicine*, 1980, *9*, 135–143.

Botvin, G., Renick, N., & Baker, E. Life skill training and smoking prevention: A one year follow up. Presented at American Public Health Association meetings, Los Angeles, November 1981.

Bradshaw, P. W. The problem of cigarette smoking and its control. *International Journal of the Addictions*, 1973, *8*, 353–371.

Brecher, E. M. *Licit and illicit drugs*. Boston: Little, Brown, 1972.

Brown, K. S., Cherry, W. H., & Forbes, W. F. The smoking habits of Canadian school children. In Canadian Council on Smoking and Health, *Proceedings of conference on student smoking*. Calgary, Alberta, October 1978.

Bynner, J. M. *The Young Smoker*. London: Her Majesty's Stationery Office, 1969.

Cameron, P. Second-hand tobacco smoke: Children's reactions: *Journal of School Health*, 1972, *42*, 280–284.

Canadian Home and School and Parent–Teacher Federation. *Students and smok-*

ing: Report of the 1971–72 Canadian School survey on cigarette smoking. Toronto, Ontario: The Canadian Home and School and Parent–Teacher Federation, 1973.

Chassin, L., Presson, C. C., Bensenberg, M., Corty, E., Olshavsky, R. W., & Sherman, S. J. Predicting adolescents' intentions to smoke cigarettes. *Journal of Health and Social Behavior*, 1981, 22(4), 445–455.

Chassin, L., Presson, C. C., Sherman, S. J., Corty, E., & Olshavsky, R. W. Self-images and cigarette smoking in adolescence. *Personality and Social Psychology Bulletin*, 1981, 7(4), 670–676.

Cherry, N., & Kiernan, K. Personality scores and smoking behavior: A longitudinal study. *British Journal of Preventive and Social Medicine*, 1976, 30, 123–131.

Clausen, J. Adolescent antecedents of cigarette smoking behavior. *Social Science and Medicine*, 1968, 1, 357–382.

Coan, R. W. Personality variables associated with cigarette smoking. *Journal of Personality and Social Psychology*. 1973, 26, 86–104.

Cook, T. D., & Flay, B. R. The persistence of experimentally induced attitude change. In L. Berkowitz (ed.), *Advances in experimental social psychology*. Vol. 11. New York: Academic Press, 1978.

Creswell, W. H., Huffman, W. J., & Stone, D. B. Youth smoking behavior characteristics and their educational implications. A report of the University of Illinois Anti-smoking Education Study. Champaign, Ill.: University of Illinois Press, 1970.

Creswell, W. H., Huffman, W. J., Stone, D. B., Merki, D. J., & Newman, I. M. University of Illinois anti-smoking education study. *Illinois Journal of Education*, 1969, 60, 27–37.

Creswell, W. H., Stone, D. B., Huffman, W. J., & Newman, I. M. Anti-smoking education study at the University of Illinois. *HSMHA Health Reports*, 1971, 86, 565–576.

Dekker, E. Youth culture and influences on the smoking behavior of young people. In *Smoking and health: Proceedings of the 3rd World Conference on Smoking and Health*. Washington, D.C.: U.S. Government Printing Office. USDHEW Publication No. (NIH) 77-1413, 1977, 381–392.

Downey, A. M., & O'Rourke, T. W. The utilization of attitudes and beliefs as indicators of future smoking behavior. *Journal of Drug Education*, 1976, 6, 283–295.

Erikson, E. H. *Childhood and society*. New York: W. W. Norton, 1963.

Evans, R. I. Smoking in children: Developing a social psychological strategy of deterrence. *Journal of Preventive Medicine*, 1976, 5, 122–127.

Evans, R. I. Smoking in children and adolescents: Psychosocial determinants and prevention strategies. In *Smoking and health: A report of the Surgeon General*. Washington, D.C.: U.S. Department of Health, Education, and Welfare, 1979.

Evans, R. I., Hansen, W. B., & Mittlemark, M. B. Increasing the validity of self-reports of smoking behavior in children. *Journal of Applied Psychology*, 1977, 62, 521–523.

Evans, R. I., Henderson, A. H., Hill, P. C., & Raines, B. E. Current psychological, social, and educational programs in control and prevention of smoking: Critical methodological review. *Atherosclerosis Reviews*, 1979, *6*, 203–245.

Evans, R. I., Rozelle, R. M., Maxwell, S. E., Raines, B. E., Dill, C. A., Guthrie, T. J., Henderson, A. H., & Hill, P. C. Social modelling films to deter smoking in adolescents: Results of a three year field investigation. *Journal of Applied Psychology*, 1981, *66*(4), 399–414.

Evans, R. I., Rozelle, R. M., Mittelmark, M. B., Hansen, W. B., Bane, A. L., & Havis, J. Deterring the onset of smoking in children: Knowledge of immediate physiological effects and coping with peer pressure, media pressure and parent modelling. *Journal of Applied Social Psychology*, 1978, *8*, 126–135.

Feather, N. T. (ed.). *Expectations and actions: Expectancy-value models in psychology*. Hillsdale, N.J.: Lawrence Elbaum Associates, 1982.

Fishbein, M. (ed.). *Readings in attitude theory and measurement*. New York: John Wiley, 1967.

Fishbein, M. Consumer beliefs and behavior with respect to cigarette smoking: A critical analysis of the public literature. In Federal Trade Commission Report to Congress: Pursuant to the Public Health Cigarette Smoking Act, for the year 1976. Washington, D.C.: U.S. Government Printing Office, 1977.

Fishbein, M., & Ajzen, I. Attitudes toward objects and predictors of single and multiple behavioral criteria. *Psychological Review*, 1974, *81*, 59–74.

Fishbein, M., & Ajzen, I. *Belief, attitude, intention and behavior: An introduction to theory and research*. Don Mills, Canada: Addison-Wesley, 1975.

Fisher, E. B. Progress in reducing smoking behavior. *American Journal of Public Health*, 1980, *70*, 678–679.

Flay, B. R. An integrative model of the attitude and behavior change process. Unpublished manuscript, University of Waterloo, 1979.

Flay, B. R. On improving the chances of mass media health promotion programs causing meaningful changes in behavior. In M. Meyer (ed.), *Health education by television and radio*. Munich: Saur, 1981.

Flay, B. R., & Best, J. A. Overcoming design problems in the evaluation of health behavior change programs. *Evaluation and the Health Professions*, 1982, *5*, 43–69.

Flay, B. R., & Cook, T. D. The evaluation of mass media prevention campaigns. In R. R. Rice & W. Paisley (eds.), *Public communication campaigns*. Beverly Hills, Calif.: Sage, 1981.

Flay, B. R., Hansen, U. B., Johnson, C. A., Alvarez, L., Sobol, D. F., Simmons, R., Kaufman, M., & Ulene, A. The USC/KABC-TV smoking prevention/cessation program: A general description. Unpublished manuscript, University of Southern California, 1982.

Glasgow, R. E., McCaul, K. D., O'Neill, H. K., Freeborn, V., & Spreier, B. Predicting adolescent smoking. Unpublished manuscript, North Dakota State University, 1981.

Goldberg, M. E., & Gorn, G. J. Some unintended consequences of TV advertising to children. *Journal of Consumer Research*, June 1978, *5*, 22–29.

Gorn, G. J., & Goldberg, M. E. The impact of television advertising on children from low income families. *Journal of Consumer Research*, September 1977, *4*, 86–88.(a)

Gorn, G. J., & Goldberg, M. E. A strategy to "demarket" cigarette smoking to teenagers: Some preliminary results. Unpublished manuscript, McGill University, 1977.(b)

Gould, L. C., Berberian, R. M., Kasl, S. V., Thompson, W. D., & Kleber, H. D. Sequential patterns of multiple drug use among high school students. *Archives of General Psychiatry*, 1977, *34*, 216–222.

Grant, R. L., & Weitman, M. Cigarette smoking and school children: A longitudinal study. In E. F. Borgatta & R. R. Evans (eds.), *Smoking, health and behavior*. Chicago: Aldine, 1968.

Green, D. E. *Teenage smoking: Immediate and long-term patterns*. Washington, D.C.: U.S. Government Printing Office, 1979.

Gritz, E. R. Smoking: The prevention of onset. The NIDA Research Monograph Series 17, *Research on Smoking Behavior*. Washington, D.C.: Department of Health, Education, and Welfare, 1977.

Gritz, E. R., & Brunswick, A. Psychosocial and behavioral aspects of smoking in women: Initiation. In *The Health Consequences of Smoking for Women: A Report of the Surgeon General*. Washington, D.C.: U.S. Government Printing Office, 1980.

Hansen, W. B., & Mittlemark, M. B. Personal versus general beliefs about consequences of smoking among youth. Unpublished manuscript, University of Southern California, 1981.

Harrison, G. N., Mohler, J. L., Lewis, L. A., & Speir, W. A., Jr. Peripheral airway function in healthy young cigarette smokers. *Lung*, 1979, *156*, 205–215.

Hartup, W. W., & Louge, M. D. Peers as models. *School Psychology Digest*, 1975, *4*:1, 11–21.

Hasenfus, J. L. Cigarette and health education among young people. *Journal of School Health*, 1971, *41*, 372–376.

Health and Welfare Canada Technical Report Series. *Smoking habits of Canadians*, Ottawa, Canada: Health and Welfare Canada, 1977.

Health and Welfare Canada Technical Report Series. *Smoking habits of Canadians*, Ottawa, Canada: Health and Welfare Canada, 1979.

Heit, P. The School Health Curriculum Project: A promising approach to the teenage smoking problem. *International Journal of Health Education*, 1978, *21*, 282–285.

Hochbaum, G. M. Public participation in medical screening programs: A sociopsychological study. U.S. Public Service Publication No. 572. Washington, D.C.: U.S. Government Printing Office, 1958.

Horn, D. Modifying smoking habits in high school students. *Children*, 1960, *1*, 63–65.

Horn, D. Behavioral aspects of cigarette smoking. *Journal of Chronic Diseases*, 1963, *16*, 383–395.

Horn, D., Courts, F. A., Taylor, R. M., & Solomon, E. S. Cigarette smoking among high school students. *American Journal of Public Health*, 1959, *49*, 1497–1511.

Hovland, C. I., Janis, I. L., & Kelly, H. H. *Communication and persuasion*. New Haven, Conn.: Yale University Press, 1953.

Hovland, C. I., Lumsdaine, A. A., & Sheffield, F. D. *Experiments on mass communication*. Princeton, N.J.: Princeton University Press, 1949.

Hranchuk, K. B., Christie, D., Hranchuk, M., & Kennedy, C. *Psycho-social aspects of cigarette smoking, 1972–76*. Ottawa, Ontario: Canadian Council on Smoking and Health, 1978.
Huntwork, D. & Ferguson, L. W. Drug use and deviation from self-concept norms. *Journal of Abnormal Child Psychology*, 1977, *5*, 53–60.
Hurd, P. D., Johnson, C. A. & Luepker, R. L. A description of the intervention strategies of an anti-smoking project conducted for junior high school students. Unpublished manuscript, University of Minnesota, 1978.
Hurd, P. D., Johnson, C. A., Pechacek, T., Bast, L. P., Jacobs, D. R., & Luepker, R. V. Prevention of cigarette smoking in seventh grade students. *Journal of Behavioral Medicine*, 1980, *3*, 15–28.
Iammarino, N., Heit, P., & Kaplan, R. School Health Curriculum Project: Long-term effects on student cigarette smoking and behavior. *Health Education*, 1980, *11*, 29–31.
Itil, T. M., Ulett, G. A., Hsu, W., Klingenberg, H., & Ulett, J. A. The effects of smoking withdrawal on quantitatively analyzed EEG. *Clinical Electroencephalography*, 1971, 2:1, 44–51.
Janis, I. L., & Mann, L. *Decision making: A psychological analysis of conflict, choice and commitment*. New York: Free Press, 1977.
Jarvik, M. E. Biological influences on cigarette smoking. In U.S. Surgeon General's Report, *Smoking and health*. Washington, D.C.: U.S. Government Printing Office, 1979.
Jarvik, M. E., Cullen, J. W., Gritz, E. R., Vogt, T. M., & West, L. J. (eds.). *Research on smoking behavior*. NIDA Research Monograph No. 17. Washington, D.C.: U.S. Department of Health, Education and Welfare, 1977, 122–148.
Jarvik, M. E., & Wong-McCarthy, W. J. Social factors in smoking. In Chien, Ching-Piao (ed.), *Sociopharmacology: Drugs in social context*. Dordrecht, Holland: D. Reidell Publishing, in press.
Jessor, R. Predicting time of onset of marijuana use: A developmental study of high school youth. *Journal of Consulting and Clinical Psychology*, 1976, *44*, 125–134.
Jessor, R. Marijuana: A review of recent psychosocial research. In R. L. Deupont, A. Goldstein, & J. A. O'Donnell (eds.), *Handbook on drug abuse*. Washington, D.C.: U.S. Government Printing Office, 1978.
Jessor, R., & Jessor, S. L. *Problem behavior*. New York: Academic Press, 1977.
Johnson, C. A. Personal communication, May 1981.
Johnson, C. A. Untested and erroneous assumptions underlying anti-smoking programs. In T. C. Coates, A. Peterson, & C. Perry (eds.), *Adolescent health: Crossing the barriers*. New York: Academic Press, in press.
Johnson, C. A., Graham, J., & Hansen, W. B. *Interaction effects of multiple risk taking behavior: Cigarette smoking, alcohol use, and marijuana use in adolescence*. Presented at the American Public Health Association Meeting, Los Angeles, November 1981.
Johnson, C. A., Luepker, R., Pechacek, T., Jacobs, D., & Hurd, P. Social factors in the prevention of smoking in seventh grade students: A follow-up experience of 1 year. Unpublished manuscript, University of Minnesota, 1979.

Johnson, C. A., Murray, D., Jacobs, D., Pechacek, T. F., Hurd, P., & Luepker, R. Effects of attitudes, normative expectations, and internality on adolescent smoking. Unpublished manuscript, University of Minnesota, 1979.

Johnston, L. D., Bachman, J. G., & O'Malley, P. M. *Drug use among American high school students, 1975–77.* National Institute on Drug Abuse. Washington, D.C.: U.S. Government Printing Office, 1977.

Johnston, L. D., Bachman, J. G., & O'Malley, P. M. *Drugs and the nation's high school students.* National Institute on Drug Abuse. Washington, D.C.: U.S. Government Printing Office, 1979.

Johnston, L. D., Bachman, J. G., O'Malley, P. M. *Highlights from student drug use in America, 1975–1981.* Washington, D.C.: U.S. Department of Health, Education, and Welfare, 1982.

Jones, E. E., Kanouse, D. E., Kelley, H. H., Nisbett, R. E., Valins, S., & Weiner, B. *Attribution: Perceiving the causes of behavior.* Morristown, N. J.: General Learning Press, 1972.

Jones, E. E., & Sigall, H. The bogus pipeline; A new paradigm for measuring affect and attitude. *Psychological Bulletin,* 1971, *76,* 349–364.

Jones, J., Piper, G. W., & Mathews, V. L. A student-directed program in smoking education. *Canadian Journal of Public Health,* 1970, *61,* 253–256.

Jöreskog, K. G., & Sörbom, D. *LISREL: Analyses of linear structural relationships by the method of maximum likelihood.* Chicago: National Education Resources, 1978.

Kales, J., Allen, C., Preston, T. A., Tan, T. L., & Kales, A. Changes in REM sleep and dreaming with cigarette smoking and following withdrawal. *Psychophysiology,* 1970, *7,* 347–348.

Kandel, D. B. Stages in adolescent involvement in drug use. *Science,* 1975, *190,* 912–914.

Kandel, D. B. (ed.). *Longitudinal research on drug use: Empirical findings and methodological issues.* Washington, D.C.: Halsted Press, 1978.

Kelson, S. R., Pullella, J. L., & Otterland, A. The growing epidemic: A survey of smoking habits and attitudes toward smoking among students in grade 7 through 12 in Toledo and Lucas County Public Schools, 1964 and 1971. *American Journal of Public Health,* 1975, *65,* 923–938.

Kozlowski, L. T. Psychosocial influences on cigarette smoking. In N. A. Krasnegor (ed.), *The behavioural aspects of smoking.* National Institute on Drug Abuse Research Monograph No. 26. Washington, D.C.: U.S. Department of Health, Education, and Welfare, 1979.(a)

Kozlowski, L. T. Psychosocial influences on cigarette smoking. In U.S. Surgeon General's Report, *Smoking and health.* Washington, D.C.: U.S. Government Printing Office, 1979.(b)

Laoye, J. A., Creswell, W. H., Jr., & Stone, D. B. A cohort study of 1205 secondary school smokers. *Journal of School Health,* 1972, *42,* 47–52.

Lefcourt, H. M. Recent developments in the study of locus of control. *Progress in Experimental Personality Research,* 1972, *6,* 1–39.

Leventhal, H., & Avis, N. Pleasure, addiction, and habit: Factors in verbal report on factors in smoking behavior. *Journal of Abnormal Psychology,* 1976, *85,* 478–488.

Leventhal, H., Brown, D., Shacham, S., & Engquist, G. Effects of preparatory information about sensations, threat of pain, and attention on cold pressor distress. *Journal of Personality and Social Psychology*, 1979, *37*, 688–714.

Leventhal, H., & Cleary, P. D. The smoking problem: A review of the research and theory in behavioural risk modification. *Psychological Bulletin*, 1981, *88*, 370–405.

Leventhal, H., & Everhart, D. Emotion, pain, and physical illness. In C. E. Izard (ed.), *Emotion and psychopathology*. New York: Plenum Press, 1979.

Levitt, E. E., & Edwards, J. A multivariate study of correlative factors in youthful cigarette smoking. *Developmental Psychology*, 1970, *2*, 5–11.

Lichtenstein, E., & Danaher, B. G. Modification of smoking behavior: A critical analysis of theory, research and practice. In M. Hersen, R. M. Eisler, & P. M. Miller (eds.), *Progress in behavior modification*. Vol. 3. New York: Academic Press, 1976.

Luepker, R. V., Pechacek, T. I., Murray, D. M., Johnson, C. A., Hurd, P., & Jacobs, D. R. Saliva thiocyanate: A chemical indicator of smoking in adolescents. *American Journal of Public Health*, 1981, *71*(12), 1320–1324.

Lutz, R. J. The functional approach to attitudes: A reconceptualization with operational implications. In J. N. Sheth (ed.), *Research in marketing*. Vol. 4. Greensich, Conn.: JAI Press, 1981.

Maiman, L. A., & Becker, M. H. The health belief model: Origins and correlates in psychology theory. In M. H. Beker (ed.), *The health belief model and personal health behavior*. Thorofare, N.J.: C. B. Slack, 1974.

Mausner, B. An ecological view of cigarette smoking. *Journal of Abnormal Psychology*, 1973, *81*, 115–126.

McAlister, A. Social and environmental influences on health behavior. *Health Education Quarterly*, 1981, 8:1, 25–31.

McAlister, A., Perry, C., Killen, J., Slinkard, L., & Maccoby, N. Pilot study of smoking, alcohol and drug abuse prevention. *American Journal of Public Health*, 1980, *70*, 719–721.

McAlister, A., Perry, C., & Maccoby, N. Adolescent smoking: Onset and prevention. *Pediatrics*, 1979, *63*, 650–658.

McGuire, W. J. Inducing resistance to persuasion. In L. Berkowitz (ed.), *Advances in experimental social psychology*. Vol. 1. New York: Academic Press, 1964.

McGuire, W. J. The nature of attitudes and attitude change. In G. Lindzay & E. Aronson (eds.), *Handbook of social psychology*. 2nd Ed. Vol. 3. Reading, Mass.: Addison-Wesley, 1969.

McGuire, W. J. Attitude change: The information processing paradigm. In C. G. McClintok (ed.), *Experimental social psychology*. New York: Holt, Rinehart and Winston, 1972.

McGuire, W. J. An information processing model of advertising effectiveness. In H. L. Davis & A. J. Silk (eds.), *Behavioral and management science in marketing*. New York: John Wiley, 1978.

McKennel, A. C. Smoking motivation factors. *British Journal of Social and Clinical Psychology*, 1970, *9*, 8–22.

McKennel, A. C. & Thomas, R. K. Adults and adolescents' smoking habits and attitudes. Government Social Survey. London: Ministry of Health, 1967.

Merki, D. J., Creswell, W. H., Stone, D. B., Huffman, W., & Newman J. The effects of two educational methods and message themes on rural youth smoking behavior. *Journal of School Health*, 1968, *38*, 448–454.

Mettlin, C. Peer and other influences on smoking behavior. *The Journal of School Health*, 1976, *16*, 529–536.

Miller, R. L., Brickman, P., & Bolan, D. Attribution versus persuasion as a means for modifying behavior. *Journal of Personality and Social Psychology*, 1975, *31*, 430–441.

Moser, R. H. The new seduction. *Journal of the American Medical Association* (editorial), 1974, *230*:11, 1564.

Murray, D. M., Johnson, C. A., Luepker, R. V., Pechacek, T. F., & Jacobs, D. R. Issues in smoking prevention research. Paper presented at the annual conference of the American Psychological Association, Montreal, September 1980.

Murray, D. M., Johnson, C. A., Luepker, R. V., Pechacek, T. F., Jacobs, D. R., & Hurd, P. Social factors in the prevention of smoking in seventh grade students: A follow-up experience of 1 year. Unpublished manuscript, University of Minnesota, 1978.

Newman, I. M. Peer pressure hypothesis for adolescent cigarette smoking. *School Health Review*, 1970, *1*, 15–18.(a)

Newman, I. M. Status configurations and cigarette smoking in a junior high school. *Journal of School Health*, 1970, *40*, 28–31.(b)

Newman, I. M., Martin, G. L., & Irwin, R. P. Attitudes of adolescent cigarette smokers. *New Zealand Medical Journal*, 1973, *79*, 237–240.

Oldendorf, W. H. Distribution of drugs to the brain. In M. E. Jarvik (ed.), *Psychopharmacology in the practice of medicine*. New York: Appleton-Century-Crofts, 1977.

Palmer, A. B. Some variables contributing to the onset of cigarette smoking in junior high school students. *Social Science and Medicine*, 1970, *4*, 359–366.

Parcel, G. S., & Meyer, M. P. Development of an instrument to measure children's health locus of control. *Health Education Monographs*, 1978, *6*, 149–159.

Pechacek, T. Modification of smoking behavior. In *Surgeon General's Report: Smoking and health*. Washington, D.C.: U.S. Department of Health, Education and Welfare, 1979.

Pederson, L. L., Baskerville, J. C., & Lefcoe, N. M. Multivariate prediction of cigarette smoking among children in grades six, seven, and eight. *Journal of Drug Education*, 1981, *11*:3, 191.(a)

Pederson, L. L., Baskerville, J. C., & Lefcoe, N. M. Prevalence of and factors related to cigarette smoking among children in grade 6. Unpublished manuscript, University of Western Ontario, 1981.(b)

Pederson, L. L., & Lefcoe, N. M. Multivariate analysis of variables related to cigarette smoking among children in grades four to six. *Canadian Journal of Public Health*, in press.

Perry, C. L. Tobacco use among adolescents: Promising trends in prevention and cessation strategies. In T. C. Coates (ed.), *Behavioral medicine: A practical handbook*. Champaign, Ill.: Research Press, in press.

Perry, C. L., & Danaher, B. G. Prevention and cessation of smoking in high school students. Unpublished manuscript, Stanford University, 1978.

Perry, C. L., Telch, M., Killen, J., & Maccoby, N. Modifying smoking behavior of teenagers: A school based intervention. *American Journal of Public Health*, 1980, *70*, 722–725.

Piper, G. W., Jones, J. A., & Mathews, V. L. The Saskatoon Smoking Project—The model. *Canadian Journal of Public Health*, 1970, *61*, 503–508.

Piper, G. W., Jones, J. A., & Mathews, V. L. The Saskatoon Smoking Study: Results of the first year. *Canadian Journal of Public Health*, 1971, *62*, 432–441.

Piper, G. W., Jones, J. A., & Mathews, V. L. The Saskatoon Smoking Study: Results of the second year. *Canadian Journal of Public Health*, 1974, *65*, 127–129.

Pomerleau, D. F. Behavioral factors in the establishment, maintenance, and cessation of smoking. In U.S. Surgeon General's Report, *Smoking and health*. Washington, D.C.: U.S. Government Printing Office, 1979.(a)

Pomerleau, D. F. Why people smoke. Current psychobiological models. In P. Davidson (ed.), *Behavioral medicine: Changing health lifestyles*. New York: Brunner-Mazel, 1979.(b)

Reynolds, C., & Nichols, R. Personality and behavioral correlates of cigarette smoking: One year follow up. *Psychological Reports*, 1976, *38*, 251–258.

Rogers, R. W. A protection motivation theory of fear appeals and attitude change. *Journal of Psychology*, 1975, *91*, 93–114.

Rosenstock, I. M. Historical origins of the health belief model. In M. H. Becker (ed.), *The health belief model and personal health behavior*. Thorofare, N.J.: C. B. Slack, 1974.

Rotter, J. B. Generalized expectancies for internal versus external control of reinforcement. *Psychological Monographs*, 1966, *80*:(1, whole No. 609).

Rush, D. Respiratory symptoms in a group of American secondary school students. The overwhelming association with cigarette smoking. *International Journal of Epidemiology*, 1974, *3*, 153–165.

Russell, M. A. H. Nicotine chewing gum as a substitute for smoking. *British Medical Journal*, 1977, *1*, 1060–1063.

Salber, E. J., Freeman, H. E., & Abelin, T. Needed research on smoking: Lessons from the Newton study. In E. F. Borgatta & R. R. Evans (eds.), *Smoking, health and behavior*. Chicago: Aldine, 1968.

Salber, E. J., Goldman, E., & Welsh, B. Smoking habits of high school students in Newton, Massachusetts. *New England Journal of Medicine*, 1961, *265*:20, 969–974.

Salber, E. J., & McMahon, B. Cigarette smoking among high school students related to social class and parental smoking habits. *American Journal of Public Health and the Nation's Health*, 1961, *51*, 1780–1789.

Salber, E. J., Welsh, B., & Taylor, S. V. Reasons for smoking given by secondary school children. *Journal of Health and Human Behavior*, 1963, *33*, 118–129.

Saltzer, E. Locus of control and the intention to lose weight. *Health Education Monographs,* 1978, *6,* 118–128.

Schacter, S. Pharmacological and psychological determinants of smoking. *Annals of Internal Medicine,* 1978, *88,* 104–114.

Schlegal, R. P., d'Avernas, J. R., & Best, J. A. Self-management and smoking cessation. A critical analysis and integrative model. Waterloo: University of Waterloo Press, 1980.

Schneider, T. W., & Van Mastrigt, L. A. Adolescent–preadolescent difference in beliefs and attitudes about cigarette smoking. *The Journal of Psychology,* 1974, *87,* 71–81.

Schuman, L. M. Patterns of smoking behavior. In M. E. Jarvik, J. W. Cullen, E. R. Gritz, T. M. Vogt, & T. J. West (eds.), *Research on smoking behavior.* NIDA Research Monograph 17. Washington, D.C.: U.S. Dept. of Health, Education and Welfare, 1977.

Sechrest, L., West, S. G., Phillips, M. A., Redner, R., & Yeaton, W. Some neglected problems in evaluation research: Strength and integrity of treatments. In L. Sechrest, S. G. West, M. A. Phillips, R. Redner & W. Yeaton (eds.), *Evaluation studies: Review annual.* Vol. 4. Beverly Hills, Calif.: Sage, 1979.

Seltzer, C. G., Friedman, G. D., & Siegelaub, A. B. Smoking and drug consumption in white, black and oriental men and women. *American Journal of Public Health,* 1974, *64,* 466–473.

Smith, G. M. Relations between personality and smoking in preadult subjects. *Journal of Consulting and Clinical Psychology,* 1969, *33,* 710–715.

Smith, G. M. Personality and smoking: A review of the empirical literature. In W. A. Hunt (ed.), *Learning mechanisms in smoking.* Chicago: Aldine, 1970.

Stanhope, J. M., & Prior, I. A. Smoking behavior and respiratory health in a teenage sample: The Rotorua Lakes Study. *New Zealand Medical Journal,* 1975, *82,* 71–76.

Stewart, L., & Livson, N. Smoking and rebelliousness: A longitudinal study from childhood to maturity. *Journal of Consulting Psychology,* 1966, *30,* 225–229.

Tennant, F. S., Jr., & Detels, R. Relationship of alcohol, cigarette and drug abuse in adulthood with alcohol, cigarette and coffee consumption in children. *Preventive Medicine,* 1976, *5,* 70–77.

Thompson, E. L. Smoking education programs, 1960–1976. *American Journal of Public Health,* 1978, *68,* 250–257.

Tomkins, S. S. Psychological model for smoking behavior. *American Journal of Public Health,* 1966, *56,* Supplement 2, 17–20.

Ulett, J. A., & Itil, T. M. Quantitative electroencephalogram in smoking and smoking deprivation. *Science,* 1969, *164,* 969–970.

U.S. Public Health Service. *Smoking and health: Report of the Advisory Committee to the Surgeon General.* Washington, D.C.: U.S. Department of Health, Education, and Welfare, 1964.

U.S. Public Health Service. *Teenage smoking: National patterns of cigarette smoking, ages 12 through 18, in 1972 and 1974.* NIH publication no. 76–931. Washington, D.C.: U.S. Department of Health, Education, and Welfare, 1976.

U.S. Public Health Service. *Smoking and health: A report of the Surgeon General*. U.S. Department of Health, Education, and Welfare, 1979.

U.S. Public Health Service. *The health consequences of smoking for women: A report of the Surgeon General*. Washington, D.C.: U.S. Department of Health and Human Services, 1980.

U.S. Public Health Service. *The health consequences of smoking: The changing cigarette. A report of the Surgeon General*. Washington, D.C.: U.S. Department of Health and Human Services, 1981.

Utech, D. A. & Hoving, K. L. Parents and peers as competing influences on the decisions of children of differing ages. Journal of Social Psychology, 1969, 78, 267–274.

Williams, T. *Summary and implications of review of literature related to adolescent smoking*. Public Health Service, Health Services and Mental Health Administration, U.S. Department of Health, Education, and Welfare, Center for Disease Control. Bethesda, Md.: National Clearinghouse for Smoking and Health, 1971.

Wohlford, P., & Giammona, S. T. Personality and social variables related to the initiation of smoking cigarettes. *Journal of School Health*, 1969, 39, 544-552.

Wong-McCarthy, W. J. Social communication functions of adolescent smoking. Research proposal, University of California at Los Angeles, 1980.

CHAPTER 7

Behavioral Treatment for Obese Children and Adolescents

Kelly D. Brownell, Ph.D.
Albert J. Stunkard, M.D.

The treatment of obesity in children is important for two reasons: (1) obese children suffer from a number of physical and psychological problems and (2) their obesity tends to persist into adult life. The obese child may demonstrate carbohydrate intolerance, increased secretion of insulin, hypercholesterolemia, elevated blood pressure, and decreased release of growth hormone (Chiumello, Del Guercio, Carnelutti, & Bidme, 1969; Clarke, Morrow, & Morse, 1970; Drash, 1973; Heald, 1971; Lauer, Conner, Leaverton, Reiter, & Clarke, 1975; Lees & Wilson, 1971; Londe, Bourgoine, Robson, & Goldring, 1971). Some atherogenic serum lipid disorders, in fact, originate in childhood (Kannel & Dawber, 1972). Adult blood pressure patterns may be predictable from childhood patterns (Zinner, Levy, & Kass, 1971). Psychological burdens include disturbed family interactions (Coates & Thoresen, 1979; Collipp, 1973; Hammar, Campbell, Campbell, Moores, Sareen, Gareis, & Lucas, 1972; Lerner & Schroeder, 1971), disapproval from peers (Lerner & Schroeder, 1971; Richardson, Goodman, & Hastorf, 1961), academic discrimination (Canning & Mayer, 1966), and poor self-image (Sallade, 1973). These physical and psychological burdens imposed upon children by obesity, while imperfectly documented, may be severe. The greater the extent of obesity, the more severe the problems.

Reprinted from Brownell, K. D., & Stunkard, A. J.: Behavioral treatment for obese children and adolescents. In Stunkard, A. J., ed.: *Obesity*. Philadelphia: W. B. Saunders Co., 1980. Used by permission.

Prevalence of Obesity in Children

Estimates of the prevalence of obesity in children vary widely, being influenced by both methodological and demographic factors. Various criteria for the determination of obesity and different methods of measurement have been employed. Social and environmental factors among the various populations studied often have not been taken into account. While it therefore is difficult to reconcile the differences in the estimates of prevalence reported, two trends nevertheless emerge. First, obesity is more prevalent among girls than among boys and, second, the prevalence of obesity increases with the increasing age of the children studied.

In two studies of young children, the prevalence of obesity in girls was reported to be ten percent (Huenemann, Hampton, Behnke, Shapiro, & Mitchell, 1974; Johnson, Burke, & Mayer, 1956). Two other studies reported prevalences of six and 15 percent (Hathaway & Sargent, 1962; Taitz, 1976). By adolescence these values all had risen. Huenemann et al. (1974) found that eight to ten percent of children in Berkeley, California were at least 20 percent overweight and five to seven percent were more than 30 percent overweight. The Ten State Nutrition Survey (Garn & Clark, 1976) reported a prevalence of ten to 30 percent for girls, and Colley (1974) reported a figure of 32 percent for girls. In each study the values for boys were lower than those for girls.

The burdens of obesity do not lighten with increasing age; obese children become obese adults. Abraham and colleagues found that more than 80 percent of people who were obese at the age of ten to 13 were obese in their 30s (Abraham, Collins, & Nordsieck, 1971; Abraham & Nordsieck, 1960). Stunkard & Burt (1967) reported on this same sample ten years later and noted that the odds against an obese child becoming a thin adult, which were four to one before adolescence, rose to 28 to one if weight reduction had not occurred by the end of adolescence.

While the physical sequelae of childhood-onset versus adult-onset obesity are not clear, the psychological consequences are more troublesome for persons with onset of obesity in childhood (Grinker, Hirsch, & Levin, 1973; Stunkard & Mendelson, 1967). Body-image disparagement occurs almost exclusively among these individuals (Stunkard & Burt, 1967; Stunkard & Mendelson, 1967), as do binge eating (bulimia) and night eating (Stunkard, 1976). It is clear that the successful treatment of obesity in childhood could yield great benefits, both physical and psychological.

Traditional programs for weight reduction in adults have been plagued by limited weight loss (Bray, 1976; Stunkard & McLaren-Hume, 1959), high dropout rates (Stunkard, 1958, 1975; Stuart, 1967; Waxler & Leef, 1969), untoward emotional reactions (Stunkard & Rush, 1974), and high

recidivism (Stunkard, 1975; Stunkard & Penick, 1979). Results of traditional approaches to the treatment of obese children have been equally discouraging (Brownell & Stunkard, 1978b; Coates & Thoresen, 1978). These
discouraging results, however, produced a climate favorable to the implementation of new methods. Behavior therapy has been subjected to extensive study since its introduction in the treatment of obesity 13 years ago.
Interestingly, studies of behavioral treatments have preceded studies of
the behaviors treated (Brownell, 1980); only recently has information on
the actual eating practices of children been elicited.

Eating, Activity, and Obesity

Treatment of obesity traditionally has involved reduction in food intake.
The fact that this course, if followed, results in weight loss leaves unanswered the question of whether obesity results from excess caloric
intake, insufficient caloric output, or both. Even though weight loss can
occur by any measure that yields a caloric deficit, it would seem logical to
produce the deficit by altering the energy balance equation on the side that
is more responsible for the obesity. We have little information about the
relative importance of caloric intake and caloric expenditure in obese
adults. We know even less about obese children. The few studies that have
examined the question are in conflict; most have serious methodological
flaws.

In 1940, Bruch reported that obese children ate more than nonobese
children, but three more recent studies found no such differences (Cahn,
1968; Lauer et al., 1975; Stephanic, Heald, & Mayer, 1959). Each study,
however, was based on parental reports, with their obvious inherent bias.

The literature on physical activity also has been inconclusive. While it is
believed widely that obese children are less active than nonobese children,
and even that inactivity may cause their obesity, most of the evidence,
again, is based on parental reports. One oft-quoted study using a more
objective measure (motion-picture sampling) did find that obese girls were
less active than nonobese girls (Bullen, Reed, & Mayer, 1964). However,
four other studies that utilized objective measures (pedometers and continuous heart-rate monitoring) failed to reveal significant differences between the activity of obese and nonobese children (Bradfield, Paulos, &
Grossman, 1971; Maxfield & Konishi, 1966; Stunkard & Peska, 1962;
Wilkinson, Parklin, Pearloom, Strang, & Sykes, 1977).

In an effort to avoid the limitations imposed by reliance on parental
reports, Waxman & Stunkard (1980) directly measured caloric intake and
energy expenditure of children in four families during meals and play in
three different settings. The subjects were four obese boys and the controls

were nonobese brothers less than two years apart in age. Nonobese class-mates served as controls for activities in school. Oxygen consumption of the subjects at four levels of activity was measured in the laboratory to permit calculation of caloric expenditure from the measures of observed activity. The obese boys consumed far more calories than the nonobese boys, but they also expended somewhat more calories. The obese boys consumed more calories (766 + 290) than did their nonobese brothers at supper (504 + 183) and far more calories (907 + 217) than their nonobese peers at lunch (500 + 386). The obese boys also ate faster (65.7 + 37.0 kcal/min) than their brothers at dinner (31.7 + 13.8 kcal/min), and much faster (103.5 + 40.9 kcal/min) than their nonobese peers at school (46.2 + 22.5 kcal/min). Time-sampled assessment of activity showed that the obese boys were far less active than their controls inside the home, slightly less active outside the home, and equally active at school. However, when these values were converted to energy expenditure per unit of activity, the picture was reversed. The obese boys expended more calories per unit of activity than did their controls. Consequently, there was no difference in caloric expenditure between obese and nonobese boys inside the home, while the obese boys actually expended more calories outside the home and in school. These findings need to be confirmed with larger samples and with studies of girls, but it is this type of intensive study that will yield information upon which successful treatment strategies can be based.

Behavioral Treatment Programs for Children

Behavioral treatments for obesity have been studied widely and have been shown to be more effective than a variety of alternative treatments for mild obesity in adults (Abrahamson, 1977; Kingsley & Wilson, 1977; Leon, 1976; Stunkard, 1975; Stunkard & Brownell, 1979; Stunkard & Mahoney, 1976; Wilson, 1978). Recent reviews have taken a cautious stance on the possible role of behavioral therapy for obesity in children (Brownell & Stunkard, 1978b; Coates & Thoresen, 1978, 1980), and studies of the efficacy of behavioral approaches to weight reduction in children have just begun.

In the past, weight-loss programs focused on what to eat. Behavioral programs widened the focus to include how to eat, on the assumption that lasting changes in eating habits must occur to produce lasting weight loss. Behavioral programs have emphasized changing the antecedents of eating (such as the salience of food cues), the rate of eating, and the consequences of eating. More detailed description of behavioral approaches may be found in Wilson (1978) and in other sources (Mahoney & Mahoney, 1976; Stuart, 1978; Stunkard & Mahoney, 1976). Specific guidelines for treating obesity in children are presented in Table 7.1.

Recently, yet another change in focus has been suggested. If obesity is viewed as a problem in adherence (Brownell, 1979; Drash, 1973), the issues of what to eat and how to eat give way to the more general question of how patients can be encouraged to adhere to a prescribed weight-loss regimen. A prescribed regimen of treatment for any disorder is useful only to the extent that the regimen is followed by the patient (Dunbar & Stunkard, 1979). If obese children and their parents are expected to follow any program of dietary change, special attention must be paid to the factors that influence how well they follow the program.

The findings from studies on behavior therapy for obese children and adolescents are summarized in Table 7.2. A detailed description of these programs follows, in which we will display the development of behavioral treatments.

Two Pilot Studies

The first systematic behavioral program for obese children was carried out in 1970 by Rivinus, Drummond, & Combrinck-Graham (1976) at the University of Pennsylvania. Ten lower-class black children (seven girls and three boys), aged eight to 13 and averaging 71 percent overweight, were selected for the program after they had continued to gain weight despite conventional treatment. During a ten-week program, the children and their mothers met weekly for two-hour sessions. The children kept records of their food intake and their adherence to the prescribed behaviors. Parents were instructed in modeling, rewards, and contracting. A novel part of the program was a weekly group supper. The children and parents sat at different tables where they were supervised in selecting low-calorie, balanced meals and were reinforced for behavioral changes such as eating slowly, self-monitoring, and putting utensils down between bites.

Nine of the ten children completed the program. The average weight loss after ten weeks was 6.2 pounds. At a four-week follow-up, four children had lost even more weight, three had maintained their weight loss, and two had regained weight to above their pretreatment levels. Considering that some developmental weight gain would be expected and that the children had been gaining weight rapidly before treatment, the results of the program were promising. Also of note was the finding that children with normal-weight mothers lost substantially more weight (11 pounds) than did children with obese mothers (2.6 pounds). At two-year follow-up, all children showed a decrease in percentage overweight. The least successful subject had gained 6.6 pounds but had grown 5.5 inches.

Table 7.1

Treatment Guidelines for Treating Obese Children and Adolescents

Obesity has multiple determinants, even within an individual. Biological, metabolic, genetic, psychological, cultural, and environmental factors may contribute to the development and/or maintenance of excess weight. In children, increased food intake may play a more important role than decreased energy expenditure; however, activity may decrease as a consequence of obesity and may promote the maintenance of obesity into adult life.

TREATMENT

Behavioral Techniques

Behavioral interventions are aimed at controlling the food environment, increasing awareness of food stimuli, structuring reinforcing consequences of appropriate eating behaviors and physical activity, and promoting attitude change.

1. Self-monitoring of food intake, calories, weight, and physical activity. It is important to emphasize habit change, but monitoring of weight loss may be more important than monitoring of specific behaviors.
2. Stimulus control concentrates on minimizing food cues, separating eating from other activities, times, and places, and preplanning.
3. Slowing the rate of eating.
4. Altering attitudes regarding eating, weight change, relapse, and so on (cognitive restructuring).
5. Increasing physical activity. This includes programmed activity (running, swimming, cycling) and routine activity (walking, climbing stairs).

Role of the Family

1. Involvement of the family can facilitate weight loss.
2. The nature of parental involvement may vary with the age of the child. With adolescents, parents should receive training, but meetings should be separate from children. As population gets younger, parents and child can meet together. With very young children, parents can meet without children.
3. Family should receive specific instructions about reinforcement, altering the food environment, and maintaining proper attitudes.
4. The family can assist in monitoring the child's eating behavior, food intake, physical activity, and weight change.
5. The family can be given nutrition education.

Role of the School

1. Peers may be helpful in a buddy system.
2. Older children can act as "sponsors" by weighing and reinforcing child.
3. Frequent weigh-ins may be useful. These can be conducted by teachers, physical education instructors, nurses, and the like.
4. The child should be reinforced for weight change, either socially with praise or tangibly with a contract that earns simple rewards.
5. A graph of weight change is useful, especially when displayed where others in the program can view it.
6. Nutrition education is important.

Table 7.2
Findings from Studies on Behavior Therapy for Obese Children and Adolescents

Study	Experimental Conditions (N)	Initial Weight Weight (lbs)	% Overweight	Weight Loss (lbs) Post	Follow Up	Comments
Rivinus et al 1976 7 girls, 3 boys; aged 8–13; low SES; black; after good conventional treatment	1. Behavioral self—control (10)	148.5	71	(10 wk) −6.2	(2 yrs) −6.7	10 weekly 2 hour sessions: weekly group supper to support modeling and monitoring for parents and children; parents learned contracting, reinforcement, and modeling; 1 subject dropped out. Children of obese mothers lost less weight.
Gross et al 1976 10 lower–middle class black girls; aged 13–17	1. Behavioral self—control (10)	179.4	39.2	(10 wk) −7.3	(12 wks) −12.5	Group meetings for 10 weeks; discussion of self—recording, calories, and social consequences of obesity.
Wheeler and Hess 1977 40 children aged 2–11 average age is 7.1	1. Behavioral self—control (14)		40.4	(8 months) change % overweight −4.1		Individual treatment in ½ hour sessions every 2 weeks for undisclosed period; less frequent meetings as children "made progress", mother and child treated to—gether; random assignment to treatment.
	2. No—treatment Control (14)	– – –	38.9	+6.3		
	3. Dropouts (12)		46.3	+3.0		

Table 7.2 (*continued*)

Study	Experimental Conditions	(N)	Initial Weight Weight (lbs)	% Overweight	Weight Loss (lbs) Post	Follow Up	Comments
Weiss 1977 11 boys, 36 girls; aged 9–18	1. Diet, no reward 2. Diet, self–reward 3. Stimulus control 4. Stimulus–control diet–self–reward 5. No–treatment control	(9) (10) (12) (9) (7)	160.8 146.0 176.3 146.3 160.6	30.7 37.5 47.2 46.2 52.1	(12 wk) −0.7 −2.7 −1.9 −2.9 +4.2	(1 yr) +9.5 +7.7 −0.3 +1.6 +18.0	Random assignment to treatment; parents told to not interfere and were not involved; 14 subjects dropped out; 12 weekly sessions of 10–15 minutes.
Kingsley and Shapiro 1977 24 boys, 16 girls from relatively affluent families aged 10–11; mothers willing to participate	1. Child only 2. Mother only 3. Mother and child together 4. Waiting list control	(10) (8) (8) (10)			(8 wk) −3.4 −3.6 −3.6 +1.9	+2.5 +2.7 − 0.3 —	Group treatment, weekly for 8 weeks; $30 deposited, earned back for attendance: treatment groups did not differ statistically and gained 0.8 pound per month during follow–up mother and child together group reported most satisfaction; mothers in mother–only group lost most weight.
Kelman et al 1979 20 girls, 6 boys; mixed SES: aged 12–15; aver– age weight −178.5 lbs. mothers willing to participate	1. Mother and child together 2. Mother and child separately 3. Child alone	(8) (7) (8)	184.0 182.2 169.3		(16 wk) −13.9 −20.5 − 6.9		3 drop –outs; 16 weekly meetings; $15 deposit from parents returned for atten– dance; $2 deposited each week from child, returned for weight loss; random assignment to treatment; stimulus control, rein– forcement, self–monitoring modeling, exercise.

Table 7.2 (continued)

Study	Experimental Conditions	(N)	Initial Weight		Weight Loss (lbs)		Comments
			Weight (lbs)	% Overweight	Post	Follow Up	
Aragona et al 1975 15 girls aged 5—10; overweight according to parents and physician	1. Response cost	(3)	105.3		(12 weeks) −9.5	(31 weeks) +7.3	Parents deposited money on a sliding scale; 25% re—funded for attendance; 25% for record keeping. 50% for weight loss; chil—dren in reinforcement group got rewards for losing weight; stimulus control, monitoring, exercise; 12 weekly meetings.
	2. Response cost plus reinforcement	(4)	105.5		−11.3	−0.7	
	3. No—treatment control	(5)	99.3		+0.9	—	
Coates et al 1978 36 adoles—cents; aged 13—17; 9% to 100% overweight	1. Daily contact, weight loss reward		179.4	36.3	(15 weeks) −15.1	(20 weeks) −16.7	15 weeks of treatment; 10 one—hour sessions using videotape, role playing, modeling, discussions, and reading. Children deposited for rewards 15 weeks of allowance or 50% of part—time earnings.
	2. Daily contact, habit change reward		160.1	36.4	− 8.4	− 7.9	
	3. Weekly contact, weight loss reward		168.5	36.4	− 4.3	− 5.9	
	4. Weekly contact, habit change reward		197.9	44.5	− 5.7	− 6.3	
Coates and Thoresen 1979 3 girls; ages 16, 16, and 15	1. Treatment subject	(1)	286	128.4	(10 weeks) −21		Intensive program; indivi—dual treatment; twice weekly meetings for 10 weeks; 5 meetings in the home with entire family; time—lagged treatments with 2 experimental subjects 1 control subject; stimulus—control, self—reward, and cognitive strategies used; rewards for weight loss and habit change.
	2. Treatment subject	(1)	194	71.4	−11.5		
	3. Control subject	(1)	215	72.9	+ 5.0		

Gross, Wheeler, & Hess (1976) reported an uncontrolled study of a similar population of ten lower-middle-class black girls, aged 13 to 17, with an average weight of 179.4 pounds. The girls met weekly for ten weeks in groups where they discussed self-recording, calories, eating patterns, and the social consequences of obesity. The average weight loss was 7.3 pounds, which had increased to 12.5 pounds at 12-week follow-up.

Two Controlled Comparisons

Behavior therapy for obese children was shown first to be more effective than no treatment by Wheeler & Hess (1976) in a study of 40 overweight children, aged two to 11. The children were assigned randomly to one of two conditions. In the behavioral condition, children and parents met in individual half-hour sessions every two weeks for an undisclosed period, and then less frequently as they "made progress." They undertook a carefully specified regimen (Stuart & Davis, 1972) that included record keeping, stimulus control, and reinforcement. Children in a control condition received no treatment.

Six children dropped out of each group, so 14 subjects remained in each condition. Those children remaining in the behavioral group decreased their average percentage overweight from 40 percent to 35 percent, while those remaining in the control group increased their average percentage overweight from 39 percent to 44 percent. While this difference was said to be statistically significant, the results are difficult to interpret because of the disparity in age among the subjects, the absence of data on actual weight loss, and the lack of follow-up.

In a more elaborate study (Weiss, 1977), 47 children (11 boys, 36 girls) aged nine to 18 and averaging 42.6 percent overweight were assigned to one of five treatment conditions:

1. Diet, no reward: Children were given an exchange diet and were awarded points for following the diet. The points were not exchanged for reinforcers.
2. Diet, self-reward: The same exchange diet was used, and the children earned points which they exchanged for self-administered reinforcers such as watching television.
3. Stimulus control: Cue control behaviors were prescribed.
4. Stimulus control, diet, self-reward: A combination of conditions 1, 2, and 3 was prescribed.
5. No-treatment control: Subjects were seen individually for 12 weekly sessions of 10 to 15 minutes each.

Parents of all children were instructed merely "not to interfere."

Fourteen of the 47 subjects dropped out of treatment, leaving 33 participants. After 12 weeks, subjects in the behavioral groups lost significantly more weight (0.7 to 2.9 pounds) than the no-treatment control group (a gain of 4.2 pounds). The treatment groups did not differ significantly. At one-year follow-up the children in the two stimulus-control groups (3 and 4) had performed significantly better (−0.3 and +1.6 pounds) than those in the other three groups, who had gained 9.5 pounds (diet, no reward), 7.7 pounds (diet, self-reward), and 18 pounds (no-treatment).

While these two studies demonstrated that behavior therapy is better than no therapy, they left many questions unanswered, one of which was the importance of parental influence.

Two Studies of the Role of the Parents

Since parents play a critical role in their child's obesity (Mayer, 1968) it seems reasonable that they also might play an important role in its treatment. Two groups have assessed this role by including parents as active members in treatment programs for their obese children. The first study showed only a trend for the parents to facilitate weight loss; the second study showed a strong effect.

Kingsley & Shapiro (1977) studied the influence of parental participation in the treatment of 24 boys and 16 girls, aged ten and 11, from relatively affluent families. The children were assigned randomly to one of four conditions:

1. Child only: Children attended treatment sessions alone and were instructed in recording food intake and stimulus-control behaviors.
2. Mother only: Mothers attended meetings alone and learned procedures identical to those in the child-only condition.
3. Mother and child together: Children and mothers attended all meetings together and received the same program as conditions 1 and 2.
4. Waiting-list control: Treatment was deferred for eight weeks.

Treatment sessions occurred weekly for eight weeks. A $30 deposit could be earned back by attending all sessions.

Figure 7.1 shows that children in the three treatment groups lost significantly more weight (3.5 pounds) during the eight-week program than did those in the no-treatment control group (who gained an average of 1.9 pounds). The three treatment conditions, however, did not differ from each other during or after treatment. During follow-up children who had been in the treatment groups gained an average of 0.8 pounds per month, approximately the expected developmental weight gain. Those in the mother-and-child-together group had regained less weight at follow-up,

Figure 7.1 Mean Weight Changes in Pounds for Overweight Children. NT = no treatment; M = mother only; C = child only; MC = mother and child together.

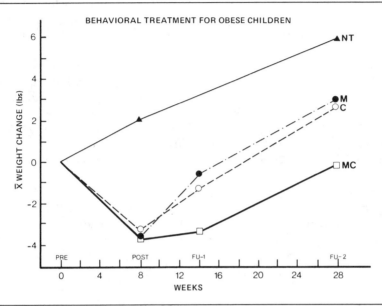

From Kingsley, R. G., & Shapiro, J. A comparison of three behavioral programs for the control of obesity in children. *Behavior Therapy*, 1977, 8, 30–36.

but the differences between this and the other groups did not reach statistical significance, perhaps because of the small sample size and the large variance in weight losses.

Kelman, Brownell, & Stunkard (1979) were successful in demonstrating the efficacy of including parents in the treatment process. Twenty-six overweight children (20 girls, six boys, aged 12 to 15, averaging 178.5 pounds in weight) were assigned randomly to one of three experimental conditions:

1. Mother and child together: Mothers and children attended all sessions together and were instructed in behavioral procedures, including self-monitoring, stimulus control, reinforcement, cognitive restructuring, family interactions, exercise management, and nutrition (Brownell, 1979).
2. Mother and child separately: Mothers and children met as two groups at the same time, but with different therapists. They received the same program as subjects in condition 1.

3. Child alone: Parents were not involved in any part of the program, and
    children received the program described for condition 1.

Treatment consisted of 16 weekly meetings, each 1.5 hours long. Parents
deposited $15 prior to treatment, with refund contingent on attendance. In
addition, each child deposited $2 per session; this was refunded if the child
lost one pound or more each week.

   As shown in Figure 7.2, after 16 weeks of treatment, those in the
child-alone group lost only 6.9 + 2.8 pounds compared to losses of 13.9 +
5.6 pounds for those in the mother-and-child-together group and 20.5 +
4.9 pounds for those in mother-and-child-separately group. Weight losses
of children in the mother-and-child-separately group were significantly
greater than losses for those in the child-alone group; losses in the mother-
and-child-together group did not differ significantly from those in the other
two groups.

   The difference in outcome between these two studies of parental participation clearly seems to result from differences in the effectiveness of the
treatments employed. The relatively large weight losses achieved in Kelman et al. (1979) permitted the effects of parental participation to be
discerned; the small weight losses achieved by Kingsley & Shapiro (1977)
did not permit such discernment.

Figure 7.2   Mean Weight Changes for Different Conditions of Parental
Involvement.

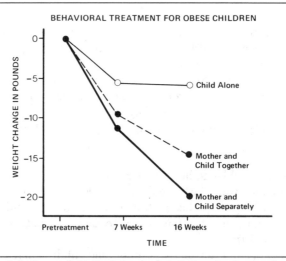

BEHAVIORAL TREATMENT FOR OBESE CHILDREN

From Kelman, S. J., Brownell, K. D., & Stunkard, A. J. The role of parental participation in
the treatment of obese adolescents. Unpublished manuscript, University of Pennsylvania,
1979.

Two Studies of Contingency Management

In contingency management, a therapeutic contract is developed whereby a child or parent earns rewards (prizes, toys, money, praise, privileges, and so on) for making predetermined changes in behavior. This procedure has been a powerful tool in the modification of childhood problems in general (Stunkard & Penick, 1979) and has shown promise in two studies with obese children.

Aragona, Cassady, & Drabman (1975) assigned 15 overweight girls (aged five to 11) to one of three conditions:

1. Response cost (deposit–refund): Parents deposited money (on a sliding scale) to be refunded in weekly portions (25 percent for attendance, 25 percent for completing charts and graphs, and 50 percent for their child's weight loss). The parents and children were instructed in stimulus control, nutrition, and exercise. The parents were given a programmed text (Patterson & Guillon, 1971), which fully explained behavioral principles, and were instructed to monitor and graph eating behavior, caloric intake, and daily weight.
2. Response cost plus reinforcement: The same terms applied here as condition 1, except each child also earned a reward. Each week the parents, child, and therapist negotiated a reward for the child that was contingent on weight loss.
3. No-treatment control.

As demonstrated in Figure 7.3, after a 12-week treatment program, the average weight losses were 9.5 pounds for those in the response-cost group (N = 4) and 11.3 pounds for those in the response-cost-plus-reinforcement group (N = 3). Those in the control group had gained 0.9 pounds (N = 5). Children in the two treatment groups lost significantly more weight than those in the control group, but the two treatment groups did not differ from each other. During a 31-week follow-up, children in both treatment groups gained weight, with the response-cost-plus-reinforcement group showing a trend toward slower rate of weight gain. At the end of 43 weeks, these subjects were still 0.7 pounds below their starting weight, while those in the response-cost group had gained 7.3 pounds. Comparisons with the control groups were no longer possible, since children in the control groups subsequently had undergone treatment.

Coates, Jeffery, Slinkard, Killen, & Danaher (1978) used a 2 × 2 factorial design to test contingency contracting and the frequency of therapist contact in 36 adolescents, aged 13 to 17 (nine to 100 percent overweight). Children were taught basic weight-loss skills in ten one-hour sessions using videotape, role-playing, modeling, group discussions, and reading assign-

Figure 7.3 Mean Weight Change in Pounds as a Function of Weeks in
Treatment for Three Experimental Groups.

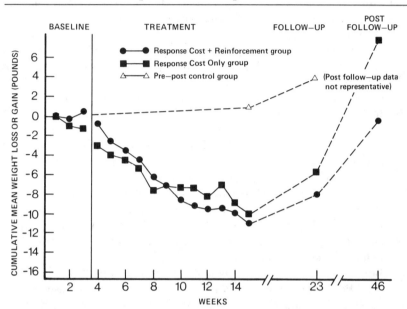

From Aragona, J., Cassady, J., & Drabman, R. S. Treating overweight children through
parental training and contingency contracting. *Journal of Applied Behavioral Analysis*, 1975,
8, 269–278.

ments. All children deposited the equivalent of 15 weeks of their allowance
or 50 percent of their estimated earnings from part-time employment.
Children in a weight-loss-reward group received refunds for losing at least
one pound each week. Children in a habit-change-reward group received
refunds for keeping calorie intake below an individually determined goal.
The frequency of contact also was manipulated by having half of the
children meet daily to receive their rewards, while the remaining half meet
weekly.

After the 15-week program, weight losses were 15.1 pounds for the
daily-contact/weight-loss-reward group, 8.4 pounds for the daily-contact/
habit-change-reward group, 4.3 pounds for the weekly-contact/weight-
loss-reward group, and 5.7 pounds for the weekly-contact/habit-change-
reward group. The daily-contact/weight-loss-reward group was the only
one to show significant change from baseline.

These two studies on contingency management show that contracting can be effective; however, weight loss does not seem to be maintained after the contract ends. Even though a great deal is known about the application of contracting to other clinical problems, little is known about its application to overweight children. The solution of these problems is likely to come from the intensive work typified by the next study.

An Intensive Evaluation

An imaginative alternative to the usual research on group treatments is the intensive single-case experiment (Hersen & Barlow, 1976) utilized by Coates & Thoresen (1979) in the study of the behavioral treatment of two obese adolescent girls and in the nonbehavioral treatment of a third. The behavioral subjects were both 16 years old and 128 percent and 71 percent overweight, while the control subject was 15 years old and 73 percent overweight.

The ten-week behavioral program included such traditional procedures as self-monitoring, stimulus control, modification of the act of eating, exercise management, and reinforcement. The children were taught cognitive restructuring to cope with self-defeating thoughts, such as, "I blew it today—I'll be fat forever." Parents were trained to support their children's use of these skills. The control subject received written descriptions of the techniques but not specific training. Intensity of contact with both behavioral and control subjects was greater than in traditional programs: The therapist met twice a week with the subjects during the ten-week program, and met once a week during the first five weeks with all family members, in the home.

This study is unique in its careful assessment of behavior change, carried out by means of time-lagged treatments and multiple-baseline observations. (The behavioral subjects received identical programs, with treatment for one subject lagged one week behind treatment for the other.) Nonparticipant observers assessed the subjects at home during dinner on four randomly selected evenings. The observers monitored the caloric value of foods in the cupboards, refrigerator, and the freezer, and during the meal they recorded the number of bites and sips per minute, the amount of time utensils were on the table, the amount of time spent talking, and the types of food eaten.

The two behavioral subjects lost 21 and 11.5 pounds, while the control subject gained 5 pounds (see Figure 7.4). Most importantly, weight loss clearly was linked to behavior change. The control subject did not change her behavior and gained weight. The treatment subjects lost weight in association with their behavior changes. Prior to treatment, one subject ate rapidly but was not exposed to high-calorie foods around the house; the

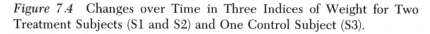

Figure 7.4   Changes over Time in Three Indices of Weight for Two
Treatment Subjects (S1 and S2) and One Control Subject (S3).

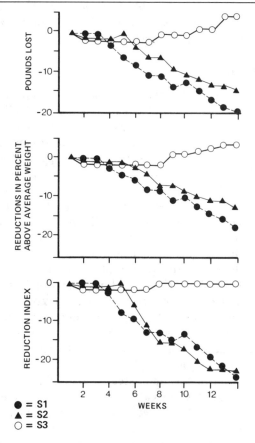

From Coates, T. J., & Thoresen, C. E. Behavior and weight changes in three obese
adolescents. *Behavior Therapy*, 1981, *12*, 383–399.

other subject showed the opposite pattern. Their respective changes in
behavior occurred only in the problem areas.

This study, noteworthy because of its careful evaluation of individual
subjects, is also one of the first to examine behavior change independent of
weight change, a valuable methdological advance (Brownell & Stunkard,
1978a; Mahoney, 1975). This kind of intensive approach may elucidate the
factors that are responsible for the large intersubject variability in behavioral programs for obesity.

Additional Factors of Potential Importance

Recent research has underscored the importance of several additional factors in the treatment of obesity; the early results are promising.

Teaching Children about Nutrition

The literature is replete with methods of imparting information about nutrition to children. There is, however, little agreement on what to teach and even less agreement on how to teach it. In one innovative study (Epstein, Masek, & Marshall, 1978), which combined nutrition education with an effort to change food preference of five- and six-year-old children, all foods were categorized into three color-coded groups—red, yellow, and green—to correspond to traffic signals. Red foods were to be avoided, yellow foods to be eaten in moderation, and green foods to be eaten freely. Children received red, yellow, and green stars according to their food selections and then were permitted to exchange the stars for inexpensive toys. Even these young children learned the system and changed their food habits in the appropriate manner.

Shoup (1975) taught eighth-grade girls to teach nutrition to elementary-school students. Not only did the younger children learn about nutrition, but the older children also increased their own knowledge. Peer influence as a vehicle for nutrition education deserves further study.

Structuring the Social Environment

The social environment has a powerful impact on eating behavior (Stunkard, 1975), particularly when eating occurs primarily in social settings, such as family dinners, school lunches, and snacks with peers.

Family intervention could become a major pathway to the control of obesity in children. The studies described earlier show that parents can have an important role in weight reduction for their children. Studies with adults demonstrate that family intervention (particularly with spouses) can greatly enhance weight loss (Brownell, Heckerman, Westlake, Hayes, & Monti, 1978; Fremouw & Zitter, 1980; Israel & Saccone, 1979; Pearce, LeBow, & Orchard, 1979; Saccone & Israel, 1978). The many complex interactions among family members must be studied before a specific program of treatment can be outlined. Studying parent–child interactions and their effect on eating and physical activity is an important area for research.

The school and the child's peers are also potential sources of social support and may be useful in combination. Peer counselors and buddy systems have been useful in school settings, and children may respond favorably to this type of influence. In one large-scale project, school personnel, family, and peers have been coordinated in a program for obese children (Kaye & Brownell, 1979). Parents and teachers have been trained in behavioral techniques and nutrition education. The children are weighed daily in the school and receive reinforcement for weight loss by teachers, school nurses, physical educaton instructors, and so forth. Some children have been assigned an older peer to act as a sponsor. The initial results of the program are favorable, and the approach appears promising.

Altering Food Preferences

The goal of nutrition education is to alter food habits in a favorable direction. The disparity of food preferences among cultures suggests that food habits can be influenced both by the availability of food and by the social environment in which food is introduced. Two important questions arise from this: (1) Can children learn preferences for nutritious foods? and (2) Can children with inappropriate preferences be weaned from problem foods? There is evidence to suggest that both are possible.

Madsen, Madsen, & Thompson (1974) used a reinforcement system to alter preferences in rural, black, economically impoverished children (mean age, six years) participating in a Head Start program. The children's normal diet was nutritionally deficient, and the children were not eating the unfamiliar but nutritious foods provided by the school. The teachers were able to double the number of children eating the unfamiliar foods by giving the children praise and pieces of sugar-coated cereal for eating the new foods. The teachers reported anecdotally that the children came to like the unfamiliar foods toward the end of the experiment. This study suffered from an unfortunate choice of reinforcers (sugared cereal), but it did show that food preferences can be altered.

Hofacker & Brenner (1976) used a modeling procedure to increase the consumption of vegetables among pediatric patients in a hospital. The children were given information about vegetables via a "vegetable parade," wherein adults, dressed as vegetables, lectured the children on the merits of individual foods. This lecture was followed by a "tasting party" at which children were encouraged to taste the vegetables. While changes in preferences were not evaluated systematically, the authors reported that the number of vegetables left uneaten decreased during the program.

Herbert-Jackson and colleagues (Herbert-Jackson, Cross, & Risley, 1977; Herbert-Jackson & Risley, 1977) have shown that preschoolers and toddlers will accept novel foods if introduced appropriately. On some days children were allowed free access to conventional foods, while on other days foods were prepared either with textured vegetable protein or with nonfat dry milk. The children ate equal amounts under both conditions, and on days when the novel foods were served, they consumed more calcium and fiber, the same amount of protein and iron, less animal fat, and fewer calories.

These studies show that food choices can be modified in school settings and that children will accept unfamiliar and nutritious foods. However, food preferences originate in the home and there have been no tests in this important setting. It is likely that the same reinforcement principles would be effective and that improved food preferences among obese children could help in weight reduction.

Program Guidelines and Conclusions

Obesity in childhood is a serious public health problem. Parents and physicians who hope that the child will "grow out of it" are likely to be disappointed; childhood obesity usually persists into adult life. The physical and psychological problems associated with obesity in children argue that the problem be taken seriously and treated aggressively.

The advent of behavior therapy for obesity has infused new promise into an area that breeds frustration in health care professionals. The conceptual framework of behavior therapy can help identify the social, environmental, physical, and cognitive determinants of obesity, and it then can help to make changes in these controlling variables. Important advances have been made in the study of obese children. Further efforts are necessary to develop a comprehensive treatment program.

Guidelines for the treatment of obese children and adolescents were presented earlier in Table 7.2. These procedures were based on findings from studies of behavior therapy with obese children and from similar studies with adults. There are three areas for intervention: the child, the family, and the school. Each can play an important role in a comprehensive weight-reduction program.

Behavioral treatment for obesity begins with self-monitoring. The child is taught to keep a careful record of food intake, calories, physical activity, and weight. This procedure increases awareness of eating patterns, portion size, and the caloric value of specific foods. Previously unnoticed patterns, such as automatic snacking, become more salient when recorded. In some cases, this procedure can alter favorably the very behavior being monitored. The records also provide parents and clinicians with information from which to establish a reinforcement program.

Stimulus control, or cue elimination, is common to nearly every behavioral program for obesity. Stimulus control consists of a series of behaviors aimed at limiting the presence of problem foods in the house and minimizing contact with high-calorie foods by keeping them out of the house. Participants are encouraged to eat at scheduled times and to avoid other activities (e.g., watching television) while eating, in order to decrease the number of times and activities associated with eating. They also are encouraged to eat at scheduled times, and to slow the act of eating, which in many cases is a rapid and automatic sequence. Instructions to put the fork down between bites and to pause during the meal help to slow eating.

Physical activity and attitude change are also important components of a weight-reduction program. Physical activity may be beneficial for the obese because of its effect on total energy expenditure, appetite, and basal metabolism. Exercise for obese children involves not only conventional sports but routine activities such as walking and using stairs. A complete description of an exercise program is presented by Brownell & Stunkard (1980). Attitude change is important to consider in cases where persons are hindered by self-defeating thoughts (e.g., "I've really blown it today. I know I'll be fat forever."). Mahoney & Mahoney (1976) thoroughly describe attitude change techniques.

Procedures for involving the family and the school in the treatment of obese children were outlined in Table 7.2. Both are potential sources of support for weight change and may provide reinforcement to the child for sustained adherence to a dietary and exercise regimen. The social relationships in these situations are complex, and involving the family and school personnel requires specific training in the principles of behavior change. Research in these areas is in its formative stages, but the results are encouraging.

Other detailed writings on this subject include those of Brownell (1979), Brownell & Stunkard (1978b), Coates & Thoresen (1978), Mahoney & Mahoney (1976), Stuart (1978), Stunkard (1975), Stunkard & Brownell (1979), and Stunkard & Mahoney (1976). Behavior therapy has great promise in the treatment of this difficult problem, but long-term maintenance of clinically significant weight loss is still elusive. It is apparent that programs must take into account differences in eating patterns (Wilson, 1978) and family situations (Brownell & Stunkard, 1978). The behavioral approach can be administered in most clinical situations and offers the most hope for controlling eating patterns of mildly to moderately obese children over the long term.

References

Abraham, S., Collins, G., & Nordsieck, M. Relationship of childhood weight status to morbidity in adults. *Public Health Report,* 1971, *86,* 273–284.

Abraham, S., & Nordsieck, M. Relationship of excess weight in children and adults. *Public Health Report,* 1960, *75,* 263–273.

Abrahamson, E. E. Behavioral approaches to weight control: An updated review. *Behavior Research and Therapy*, 1977, *15*, 355–364.

Aragona, J., Cassady, J., & Drabman, R. S. Treating overweight children through parental training and contingency contracting. *Journal of Applied Behavioral Analysis*, 1975, *8*, 269–278.

Bradfield, R., Paulos, J., & Grossman, H. Energy expenditure and heart rate of obese high school girls. *American Journal of Clinical Nutrition*, 1971, *24*, 1482–1486.

Bray, G. A. *The obese patient*. Philadelphia: W. B. Saunders, 1976.

Brownell, K. D. Obesity and adherence to behavioral programs. National Institute on Drug Abuse Research Monograph 25. Washington, D.C.: U.S. Government Printing Office, June 1979.

Brownell, K. D. Behavior therapy for weight control: A treatment manual. Unpublished manuscript, University of Pennsylvania, 1979.

Brownell, K. D. Assessment in the treatment of eating disorders. In D. H. Barlow (ed.), *Assessment of adult disorders*. New York: Guilford Press, 1980.

Brownell, K. D., Heckerman, C. L., Westlake, R. J., Hayes, S. C., & Monti, P. M. The effect of couples training and partner cooperativeness in the behavioral treatment of obesity. *Behaviour Research and Therapy*, 1978, *16*, 323–333.

Brownell, K. D., & Stunkard, A. J. Behavior therapy and behavior change: Uncertainties in programs for weight control. *Behaviour Research and Therapy*, 1978, *16*, 301. (a)

Brownell, K. D., & Stunkard, A. J. Behavioral treatment of obesity in children. *American Journal of Diseases in Children*, 1978, *132*, 403–412. (b)

Brownell, K. D., & Stunkard, A. J. Physical activity in the development and control of obesity. In A. J. Stunkard (ed.), *Obesity*. Philadelphia: Saunders, 1980.

Bruch, H. Obesity in childhood. Part III. Physiological and psychological aspects of food intake of obese children. *American Journal of Diseases in Children*, 1940, *59*, 739–748.

Bullen, B. A., Reed, R. B., & Mayer, J. Physical activity of obese and non-obese adolescent girls appraised by motion picture sampling. *American Journal of Clinical Nutrition*, 1964, *14*, 211–233.

Cahn, A. Growth and caloric intake of heavy and tall children. *Journal of American Dietetic Association*, 1968, *53*, 476–480.

Canning, H., & Mayer, J. Obesity—its possible effect on college acceptance. *New England Journal of Medicine*, 1966, *275*, 1172–1174.

Chiumello, G., Del Guercio, M. J., Carnelutti, M., & Bidme, G., Relationship between obesity, chemical diabetes, and beta pancreatic function in children. *Diabetes*, 1969, *18*, 238–243.

Clarke, R. P., Morrow, S. B., & Morse, E. H. Interrelationships between plasma lipids, physical measurements, and body fatness of adolescents in Burlington, Vermont. *American Journal of Clinical Nutrition*, 1970, *23*, 754–763.

Coates, T. J., Jeffery, R. W., Slinkard, L. A., Killen, J. D., & Danaher, B. G. Frequency of contact and monetary incentives in weight reduction with adolescents. Paper presented at the annual meeting of the Association for the Advancement of Behavior Therapy, Chicago, 1978.

Coates, T. J., & Thoresen, C. E. Treating obesity in children and adolescents: A review. *American Journal of Public Health*, 1978, *68*, 143–151.

Coates, T. J., & Thoresen, C. E. The efficacy of a multicomponent self-control program in modifying the eating habits and weight of three obese adolescents. Unpublished manuscript, Stanford University, 1979.

Coates, T. J., & Thoresen, C. E. Obesity among children and adolescents: the problem belongs to everyone. In B. Lahey & A. E. Kazdin (eds.), *Advances in clinical child psychology*. New York, Plenum Press, 1980.

Coates, T. J. & Thoresen, C. E. Behavior and weight changes in three obese adolescents. *Behavior Therapy*, 1981, *12*, 383–399.

Colley, J. R. T. Obesity in school children. *British Journal of Social and Preventative Medicine*, 1974, *28*, 221–225.

Collipp, P. J. Nutrition of the fetus, infant, and child. *American Journal of Diseases in Children*, 1973, *126*, 558–560.

Drash, A. Relationship between diabetes mellitus and obesity in the child. *Metabolism*, 1973, *22*, 337–344.

Dunbar, J. M., & Stunkard, A. J. Adherence to diet and drug regimens. In R. Levy, B. Rifkind, B. Dennis, & N. Ernst (eds.), *Nutrition, lipids and coronary heart disease*. New York: Raven Press, 1979.

Epstein, L. H., Masek, B. J., & Marshall, W. R. A nutritionally based school program for control of eating in obese children. *Behavior Therapy*, 1978, *9*, 766–778.

Fremouw, W. J., & Zitter, R. E. Individual and couple behavioral contracting for weight reduction and maintenance. *Behavior Therapist*, 1980, *3*, 15–16.

Garn, S. M., & Clark, D. C. Trends in fatness and the origins of obesity. *Pediatrics*, 1976, *57*, 443–456.

Grinker, J., Hirsch, J., & Levin, B. The affective response of obese patients to weight reduction: A differentiation based on age at onset of obesity. *Psychosomatic Medicine*, 1973, *35*, 57–63.

Gross, I., Wheeler, M., & Hess, R. The treatment of obesity in adolescents using behavioral self-control. *Clinical Pediatrics*, 1976, *15*, 920–924.

Hammar, S. L., Campbell, M. M., Campbell, V. A., Moores, N. L., Sareen, C., Gareis, F. J., & Lucas, B. An interdisciplinary study of adolescent obesity. *Journal of Pediatrics*, 1972, *80*, 373–383.

Hathaway, M. L., & Sargent, D. W. Overweight in children. *Journal of American Dietetic Association*, 1962, *40*, 511–515.

Heald, F. P. Biochemical aspects of juvenile obesity. *Practitioner*, 1971, *206*, 223–226.

Herbert-Jackson, E., Cross, M. Z., & Risley, T. R. Milk types and temperature: What will young children drink? *Journal of Nutrition Education*, 1977, *9*, 76–79.

Herbert-Jackson, E., & Risley, T. R. Behavioral nutrition: Consumption of foods of the future by toddlers. *Journal of Applied Behavioral Analysis*, 1977, *10*, 407–414.

Hersen, M., & Barlow, D. H. *Single case experimental designs: Strategies for studying behavior change*. New York: Pergamon Press, 1976.

Hofacker, R., & Brenner, N. Vegetable parade persuades children to try new foods. *Journal of Nutrition Education*, 1976, *8*, 21–24.

Huenemann, R. L., Hampton, M. C., Behnke, A. R., Shapiro, L. R., & Mitchell, B. W. *Teenage nutrition and physique*. Springfield, Ill.: Charles C Thomas, 1974.

Israel, A. C., & Saccone, A. J. Follow-up effects of choice of mediator and target of reinforcement on weight loss. *Behavior Therapy*, 1979, *10*, 260–265.

Johnson, M. L., Burke, B. S., & Mayer, J. Relative importance of inactivity and overeating in the energy balance of obese high school girls. *American Journal of Clinical Nutrition*, 1956, *4*, 37–44.

Kannel, W. B., & Dawber, T. R. Atherosclerosis as a pediatric problem. *Journal of Pediatrics*, 1972, *80*, 544–554.

Kaye, F., & Brownell, K. D. A comprehensive school-based program for the treatment of obese elementary school children. Unpublished manuscript, University of Pennsylvania, 1979.

Kelman, S. J., Brownell, K. D., & Stunkard, A. J. The role of parental participation in the treatment of obese adolescents. Unpublished manuscript, University of Pennsylvania, 1979.

Kingsley, R. G., & Shapiro, J. A comparison of three behavioral programs for control of obesity in children. *Behavior Therapy*, 1977, *8*, 30–36.

Kingsley, R. G., & Wilson, G. T. Behavior therapy for obesity: A comparative investigation of long-term efficacy. *Journal of Consulting and Clinical Psychology*, 1977, *45*, 288–298.

Lauer, R. M., Conner, W. E., Leaverton, P. E., Reiter, M. A., & Clarke, W. R. Coronary heart disease risk factors in school children. *Journal of Pediatrics*, 1975, *86*, 697–700.

Lees, R. S., & Wilson, D. E. The treatment of hyperlipidemia. *New England Journal of Medicine*, 1971, *284*, 186–194.

Leon, G. R. Current directions in the treatment of obesity. *Psychological Bulletin*, 1976, *83*, 557–578.

Lerner, R. M., & Schroeder, C. Kindergarten children's active vocabulary about body build. *Developmental Psychology*, 1971, *5*, 179.

Londe, S., Bourgoine, J. J., Robson, A. M., Goldring, D. Hypertension in apparently normal children. *Journal of Pediatrics*, 1971, *78*, 569–577.

London, A. J., & Schreiber, E. D. A controlled study of the effects of group discussions and an anorexiant in outpatient treatment of obesity. *Annals of Internal Medicine*, 1966, *65*, 80–92.

Madsen, C. H., Madsen, C. K., & Thompson, F. Increasing rural Head Start children's consumption of middle-class meals. *Journal of Applied Behavior Analysis*, 1974, *7*, 257–262.

Mahoney, M. J. The obese eating style: Bites, beliefs, and behavior modification. *Addictive Behavior*, 1975, *1*, 47–53.

Mahoney, M. J., & Mahoney, K. *Permanent weight control: A total solution to the dieter's dilemma*. New York: W. W. Norton, 1976.

Maxfield, E., & Konishi, F. Patterns of food intake and physical activity in obesity. *Journal of American Dietetic Association*, 1966, *49*, 406–408.

Mayer, J. *Overweight: Causes, cost, and control*. Englewood Cliffs, N.J.: Prentice-Hall, 1968.

Patterson, G. R., & Guillon, M. E. *Living with children: New methods for parents and teachers*. Champaign, Ill.: Research Press, 1971.

Pearce, J. W., LeBow, M. D., & Orchard, J. The role of spouse involvement in the behavior treatment of obese women. Paper presented at the annual meeting of the Canadian Psychological Association, Montreal, Quebec, 1979.

Richardson, S. A., Goodman, N., & Hastorf, A. H. Cultural uniformity in reaction to physical disabilities. *American Sociological Review*, 1961, *26*, 241–247.

Rivinus, T. M., Drummond, T., & Combrinck-Graham, L. A group-behavior treatment program for overweight children: The results of a pilot study. *Pediatric Adolescent Endocrinology*, 1976, *1*, 212–218.

Saccone, A. J., & Israel, A. C. Effects of experimenter versus significant other-controlled reinforcement and choice of target behavior on weight loss. *Behavior Therapy*, 1978, *9*, 271–278.

Sallade, J. A comparison of the psychological adjustment of obese and non-obese children. *Journal of Psychosomatic Research*, 1973, *17*, 89–96.

Shoup, E. W. Teens teach children nutrition. *Journal of Nutrition Education*, 1975, *7*, 107–108.

Stefanic, P. A., Heald, F. P., & Mayer, J. Caloric intake in relation to energy output of obese and nonobese adolescent boys. *American Journal of Clinical Nutrition*, 1959, *7*, 55–62.

Stuart, R. B. Behavioral control of overeating. *Behavior Research and Therapy*, 1967, *5*, 357–365.

Stuart, R. B. *Act thin, stay thin*. New York: W. W. Norton, 1978.

Stuart, R. B., & Davis, B. *Slim chance in a fat world: Behavioral control of obesity*. Champaign, Ill.: Research Press, 1972.

Stunkard, A. J. The management of obesity. *New York State Journal of Medicine*, 1958, *58*, 79–87.

Stunkard, A. J. From explanation to action in psychosomatic medicine: The case of obesity. *Psychosomatic Medicine*, 1975, *37*, 195–236.

Stunkard, A. J. *The Pain of Obesity*. Palo Alto, Calif.: John Bull, 1976.

Stunkard, A. J., & Brownell, K. D. Behavior therapy and self-help programs for obesity. In J. F., Munro (ed.), *The treatment of obesity*. London, MTP Press, 1979.

Stunkard, A. J., & Burt, V. Obesity and the body image. Part II. Age at onset of disturbances in the body image. *American Journal of Psychiatry*, 1967, *123*, 1443–1447.

Stunkard, A. J., & Mahoney, M. J. Behavioral treatment of eating disorders. In H. Leitenberg (ed.) *The handbook of behavior modification*. Englewood Cliffs, N.J.: Prentice-Hall, 1976.

Stunkard, A. J., & McLaren-Hume, M. The results of treatment for obesity. *Archives of Internal Medicine*, 1959, *103*, 79–85.

Stunkard, A. J., & Mendelson, M. Obesity and body image. Part I. Characteristics of disturbances in the body image of some obese persons. *American Journal of Psychiatry*, 1967, *123*, 1296–1300.

Stunkard, A. J., & Penick, S. B. Behavior modification in the treatment of obesity: The problem of maintaining weight loss. *Archives of General Psychiatry*, 1979, *36*, 801–806.

Stunkard, A. J., & Pestka, J. The physical activity of obese girls. *American Journal of Diseases of Children*, 1962, *103*, 812–817.

Stunkard, A. J., & Rush, A. J. Dieting and depression reexamined: A critical review of reports of untoward responses during weight reduction for obesity. *Annals of Internal Medicine*, 1974, *81*, 526–533.

Taitz, L. S. Infantile overnutrition among artificially fed infants in the Sheffield region. *British Medical Journal*, 1976, *1*, 315–316.

Waxler, S. H., & Leef, M. F. Obesity—Doctor's dilemma. *Geriatrics*, 1969, *24*, 98–106.

Waxman, M., & Stunkard, A. J. Caloric intake and expenditure of obese children. *Journal of Pediatrics*, 1980, *96*, 187–193.

Weiss, A. R. A behavioral approach to the treatment of adolescent obesity. *Behavior Therapy*, 1977, *8*, 720–726.

Wheeler, M. E., & Hess, K. W. Treatment of juvenile obesity by successive approximation control of eating. *Journal of Behavior Therapy and Experimental Psychiatry*, 1976, *7*, 235–241.

Wilkinson, P., Parklin, J., Pearloom, G., Strang, H., & Sykes, P. Energy intake and physical activity in obese children. *British Medical Journal*, 1977, *1*, 756.

Wilson, G. T. Methodological considerations in treatment outcome research on obesity. *Journal of Consulting and Clinical Psychology*, 1978, *46*, 687–702.

Zinner, S. H., Levy, P. S., & Kass, E. H. Familial aggregation of blood pressure in children. *New England Journal of Medicine*, 1971, *284*, 401–408.

CHAPTER **8**

Compliance in Pediatric Populations: A Review

Jacqueline Dunbar, Ph.D.

Research on patient compliance with health care regimens has grown exponentially over the past ten to 15 years. Most of this research has been directed to adults in outpatient settings. Less attention has been given to compliance in the pediatric population, where the concern is with parents' management of their children's health care prescriptions. This chapter reviews the state of the art in pediatric compliance, including information on the compliance rates for chronic and acute conditions, factors that have been associated with pediatric compliance, and the results of intervention studies. Suggestions for future research are offered.

Attention to compliance is important in pediatric populations, as in adult populations, for at least three reasons. The first of these concerns research on the efficacy of treatment. Compliance must be attended to if one is to increase the sensitivity of these studies. The efficacy of the treatment, the safety of the treatment, and the incidence of side-effects cannot be assessed unless compliance with the experimental regimen is accounted for. This is the case in both the study of medication treatments as well as behavioral treatments. Second, compliance also must be accounted for if one is to evaluate treatment efficacy in the clinical situation. It is not possible to determine if the advice or prescription offered the patient is appropriate if the patient does not comply. Third, compliance must be attended to and encouraged if one is to obtain maximum therapeutic benefit. No treatment will work if the patient is not willing to adhere to it.

Definitions of Compliance

Unfortunately, many studies and many clinicians still do not address compliance adequately. A major reason for this is the lack of standard definitions. The approach to defining compliance varies from study to study and clinician to clinician; however, these definitions tend to fall within one of three categories. The first of these categories expresses the quantity of the regimen that has been carried out. This usually is expressed as a percent or as a ratio. The second type of definition clusters persons into various compliance categories; that is, patients may be good, moderate, poor, or noncompliers. The third type of definition is an index of compliance, which basically gives each person an overall score based on a number of health care behaviors.

Percentage Definition

Probably the most informative definition is the percentage of the regimen actually carried out. This allows the reader to draw his own conclusions regarding acceptable levels of compliance. The percentage definition facilitates comparisons across studies, regimens, or populations, allowing the reader to examine the range or distribution of compliance levels for a given drug or a given intervention program. Interestingly, of 23 medication studies in the pediatric area that were reviewed, none reported data on the percentage of the regimen completed by patients. Three of the studies (13 percent) reported using a pill or liquid count to determine the percentage adherence to a medication, but then simply reported the percentage of children who fell into some qualitative category. As well, these studies used different quantitative criteria for placing patients in the qualitative category of "good complier."

For example, Buchanan & Mashigo (1977) used a relatively stringent criterion for classifying patients as good adherers. Two hundred South African pediatric patients were visited in their homes, unannounced, five to eight days after a visit to the hospital physician. During this visit, the amount of medication taken was assessed. Patients who had consumed 100 percent of their regimen were classified as good adherers. Persons with any remaining medication, which should have been taken, were considered noncompliant.

Arnhold, Adebonojo, Callas, Callas, Carte, & Stein (1970) were somewhat less stringent but, like Buchanan & Mashigo (1977), determined quantitatively the amount of medication that was consumed in a group of 104 patients on antibiotics. Again, a home visit was made to patients shortly after a visit to the physician. During the course of the visit, the amount of remaining medication was counted and a determination was made of the percent of compliance. These figures were not reported. Instead, patients were categorized as compliers or noncompliers and the percentage of compliant patients was reported. The patient was judged to be compliant if the medication remaining did not deviate from the calculated amount by more than one day's dose. As most of the prescriptions were for five- to ten-day courses of treatment, this meant that patients needed to take 80 percent to 90 percent of their doses to be classified as good adherers.

In the third study, Lima, Nazarian, Charney, & Lahti (1976) set a 70 percent adherence rate as a minimum for good adherence. One hundred and fifty-eight patients on antibiotic therapy were visited at home, and the amount of medication remaining was counted. As in the preceding two studies, the means of the distributions were not reported. The percentage of patients who fell into the category of good compliance was 24. Thus, we not only find limited use of the quantitative definition of compliance in pediatric literature, we find that even in those cases where a quantitative definition could be reported, it rarely is.

Category Definition

The most common type of definition in the pediatric studies is the category definition. Indeed, if we include the three studies previously reported, 87 percent of the 23 studies reviewed used this type of definition. What is meant here is the classification of patients into various qualitative groups, that is, good adherers, moderate adherers, poor adherers, nonadherers, and so forth.

The category definition is problematic for several reasons. In most cases, there is not a scientific basis for determining eligibility for the good-compliance category. For the majority of regimens prescribed for patients, there is no knowledge of how much that regimen needs to be carried out in order to achieve a good therapeutic outcome. If biological measures are utilized to classify persons, then individual differences in metabolism can lead persons with different medication-taking behaviors to be grouped together. Conversely, patients with similar medication-taking behaviors or compliance rates might be placed into different categories. Given a lack of scientific basis for determining cutoff points for various categories and the problems in using biological assays to do this, most researchers have utilized arbitrary cutoff points to classify patients. The use of arbitrary cutoff points, however, limits comparisons across studies. In the pediatric studies reviewed, several cutoff points or definitions of compliance were used. Buchanan & Mashigo (1977) required the person to be 100 percent compliant, that is, to have no medication remaining on a certain date, to be classified as a good adherer or good complier. Arnhold et al. (1970) allowed no more than one day's deviation from the prescribed antibiotic regimen. Lima et al. (1976) required that at least 70 percent of an antibiotic regimen must have been consumed. Determinations of percentage of medication consumed with arbitrary standards for classifying the person as a good adherer was the way such categorization was made.

Three other researchers examined antimicrobial activity in urine as an estimation of patient compliance with antibiotic therapy. Again, different cutoff points were set. Using a technique described by Markowitz & Gordis (1968), Colcher & Bass (1972) examined 300 patients with streptococcal pharyngitis who were on antibiotic therapy. These researchers required patients to have a positive urine test for antimicrobial activity on the ninth day of treatment to be classified as good adherers. There was no information on the percentage of medication consumed by these patients.

In the second study, Meyers, Dolan, & Mueller (1975) examined 61 patients with cystic fibrosis who were on antibiotic therapy. In this case, the researchers required that patients have 100 percent of five urine tests positive for antimicrobial activity over a two-month time period in order to be classified as good adherers. Unlike the Colcher & Bass study (1972), which classified patients as either compliant or noncompliant based on a single measure, Meyers et al. (1975) classified patients as compliant if 100 percent of the tests were positive, intermediate if 70 percent to 99 percent of the samples were positive, and poor if less than 70 percent of the samples showed antimicrobial activity.

Gordis, Markowitz, & Lilienfeld (1969a) also examined a series of urine specimens over a five-month time period. In 136 children and adolescents on daily penicillin prophylaxis for rheumatic fever, 75 percent of random weekly urine specimens over a five-month time period had to be positive for antimicrobial activity for the child to be classified as a good complier. Children were classified as intermediate if 26 percent to 74 percent of the urine specimens were positive. For those patients for whom 25 percent or less of the specimens evidenced antimicrobial activity, the classification was as a noncomplier.

Thus, across these three studies, "good compliance" varied from antimicrobial activity in 100 percent of urine samples to activity in more than 75 percent of urine samples; "intermediate compliance" varied from between 70 percent and 99 percent to between 26 percent and 74 percent. The intermediate group in one study would have been classified as good adherers in the second study. One study classified as poor compliers all persons with 99 percent or fewer urine specimens demonstrating antimicrobial activity; a second gave this rating at the level of 70 percent or less of the urine specimens; and a third study, at less than 25 percent. The problem of comparing across studies when arbitrary classifications are utilized is quite evident. Indeed, there are nearly as many definitions of good, intermediate, and poor compliance as there are investigators categorizing compliant behavior. It is important to keep this fact in mind when one considers the rates of noncompliance in the pediatric population.

Index Definition

The third type of definition utilized in the pediatric studies is the index
definition of compliance. Essentially, the index of compliance sums across
a set of behaviors or regimens that the patient is expected to carry out.
These figures are grouped to form a single composite compliance score.
Three studies, or 13 percent of those reviewed, utilized this type of
definition, reporting the percentage of the sample that was deemed compliant. Litt, Cuskey, & Rudd (1980), in a study of compliance with contraceptive therapy among adolescents, combined three behaviors to evaluate compliance. These behaviors included (1) returning for follow-up
appointments, (2) the self-reported consistent use of a diaphragm, (3)
checking the IUD string, (4) not missing more than two pills per month,
and (5) not becoming pregnant. Francis, Korsch, & Morris (1969), in the
classic study of doctor–patient communication, combined medication consumption, adherence to various other treatments, diet, return for follow-
up appointments, and compliance with any other advice to form a single
composite compliance score. Similarly, Becker, Drachman, & Kirscht
(1972), in a test of the health-belief model with pediatric patients, combined the mother's knowledge of the name of the medication that was
prescribed to her child, with her knowledge of the number of times a day it
was to be given, her knowledge of the follow-up appointment date, the
actual administration of the medication, and keeping the follow-up
appointment.

As may be evident, there are many problems with the index type of
definition. While it measures compliance to a whole treatment program, it
obscures the individual components of the regimen. One does not have a
sense of how these individual components are rated to make up the final
composite score. Further, it is not known whether knowledge, appointment keeping, medication taking, diet adherence, or any other aspects of
the treatment program are sufficiently related to allow them to be treated
as elements of the same behavior, that is, compliance. Bearing in mind
these definitional problems, let us turn to an examination of the extent of
the compliance problem in the pediatric population.

Extent of the Compliance Problem

In the adult population, compliance problems are found in 25 percent to 80
percent of patients. The rates look no better in the pediatric group. In a
recent review by Litt & Cuskey (1980), overall noncompliance rates were
estimated at 50 percent, with a range of 20 percent to 80 percent. The rates
found in the studies reviewed here tend to be somewhat lower. Among

acute conditions, the percentage of the population that is judged compliant ranges from 18 percent to 58 percent (see Table 8.1). In each of the studies reviewed, patients were on short-term antibiotic therapy. Fifty-eight percent of patients with streptococcal pharyngitis were found to be compliant with antibiotic therapy, based on a urine assay for antimicrobial activity conducted by Colcher & Bass (1972). A similar rate of 51 percent was reported by Arnhold et al. (1970), who used a home pill count for patients on antibiotics for a variety of problems. Becker et al. (1972) reported 40 percent of patients to be compliant with antibiotic prescriptions for otitis media, based on unannounced urine assays. Less than one-fourth of persons were judged to be compliant by Fink, Malloy, Cohen, Greycloud, & Martin (1969) and Lima et al. (1976), based on interview or home pill count, respectively. The rates range from 42 percent to more than 75 percent of patients judged noncompliant. The rates are somewhat better in preventive short-term regimens, that is, immunization of newborns. At least one study, Barkin, Barkin, & Roth (1977) reported 78 percent of parents were compliant with recommendations for newborn immunizations. This seems to be in keeping with other national figures showing that approximately 75 percent of one year olds are reported to have received their immunizations.

The rates on chronic conditions are similar, ranging from 11 percent to 88 percent in the studies reviewed in this chapter. Where they are separated out, in chronic conditions (unlike acute conditions), adolescents seem to do less well than younger children, and where biological measures are contrasted with indirect measures, the biological measures tend to show

Table 8.1
Extent of Medication Compliance in Acute Conditions: Pediatric Population

Author/Year	% Compliant	Compliance Measure
General problems		
Arnhold et al., 1970	51	Home pill count
Fink et al., 1969	18	Interview
Lima et al., 1976	24	Home pill count
Otitis media		
Becker et al., 1972	40.1	Unannounced urine sampling
Streptococcal pharyngitis		
Colcher & Bass, 1972	58	Urine sampling

lower rates. With the exception of the high rates of compliance among children with cystic fibrosis on antibiotic therapy and children on chemotherapy, the range of compliance appears similar across chronic disease conditions (see Table 8.2).

As with short-term therapies, compliance rates tend to vary with the measurement used. For example, in patients on long-term prophylactic penicillin the proportion of patients deemed compliant across studies ranged from 36 percent, using randon urine assay as the measure of compliance, through 50 to 57 percent, using clinical judgement, and 57.6 to 67.8 percent using routine urine assays, to as high as 82.8 to 87.9 percent using interview as the method of assessing compliance. It is not clear from the table what might contribute to the differences found with age, although it is possible that the investigators were measuring parent compliance in children and self-compliance in adolescents.

Table 8.2
Extent of Medication Compliance in Chronic Conditions: Pediatric Population

Author/Year	% Compliant	Compliance Measure
Asthma		
Eney & Goldstein, 1976	11	Saliva
Sublett et al., 1979	24.5	Serum
Radius et al., 1978	66.3	Serum
Cancer		
Smith et al., 1979	41 (adolescents)	Urine sample
	82 (children)	
Contraception		
Litt, Cuskey, & Rudd, 1980	44.6	Interview
Cystic Fibrosis		
Meyers et al., 1975	80	Urine sample
Epilepsy		
Dawson & Jamieson, 1971	25	Serum
Freiman & Buchanan, 1978	25–58	Serum
Rheumatic Fever		
Gordis et al., 1969b	57.6–67.8	Urine sample
	82.8–87.9	Interview
Gordis et al., 1969a	36	Random urine sample
Wood et al., 1964	50–57	Clinical judgment

The compliance rates for children with both acute and chronic conditions are no better than those rates seen for adults. One has to keep in mind, in interpreting these figures, that the definitions for good adherence vary from study to study and, indeed, may vary considerably. Thus we may not be talking about comparable levels of behavioral performance among these patients. Further, the proportion of persons who are judged compliant seems to vary to some extent with the type of measure utilized by the researcher. It seems appropriate, then, to turn to an examination of the various measurement strategies available to the clinician and the researcher interested in compliance in the pediatric population.

Measurement of Compliance

Six types of measures currently are available for the assessment of compliance. These include the biological indices, clinician ratings, self-report, pill or bottle counts, direct observation, and some form of mechanical monitoring.

Biological indices were the most commonly used form of measurement in the pediatric studies reviewed. These form the only direct measure of compliance. These indices include such things as (1) urine assays to determine antimicrobial activity as a function of the ingestion of antibiotics, (2) serum levels of phenytoin or other drugs, and (3) the detection of theophylline in the patient's saliva. While these measures give direct indication of whether or not the patient has taken medication, they do have three major problems in the determination of compliance. In the first case, there are individual differences in the absorption and metabolism of drugs. Thus, absence of therapeutic levels may be due either to the fact that the patient did not consume the medication or to the fact that the patient has some abnormal metabolism of the drug. Certainly, the biological indices do not measure degree of compliance. They simply indicate whether or not some amount of medication was consumed. One does not know if the patient took all of the prescription or a part of it. Further, the biological indices do not measure compliance over time. These measures only give information on whether or not the patient took any medication within some relatively short time period prior to the assessment.

These biological indices should not be confused with therapeutic outcome, which does not constitute a measure of patient compliance. Compliance is certainly a mediator of therapeutic outcome; however, there is not necessarily a direct correspondence between the two. The patient may be on inappropriate therapy or an inadequate dose of therapy, complying well and still not achieving the therapeutic outcome. Similarly, the patient may be getting an adequate response from poor levels of compliance due to his own individual responsiveness to treatment or to overdosing in the prescription.

The second type of measure is clinical rating or clinical judgment. This is probably the poorest measure of compliance. This method was used in only one of the compliance studies cited (Wood, Feinstein, Taranta, Epstein, & Simpson, 1964). Much of the literature suggests that we as clinicians do no better than chance at determining which patient is or is not compliant. Indeed, it probably would be best if this measure were not utilized at all.

The third type of measure that can be utilized in compliance assessment is self-report, either via self-monitoring or interview. Self-monitoring was not utilized in any of the pediatric studies reviewed, but it is a measure that offers a wealth of information. The diary or calendar can be utilized for recording compliance episodes. In the case of the adolescent or older child, the child may be able to carry out this responsibility. For the younger child, this may be a task for the parent. Because self-monitoring can be reactive, care must be taken to maintain its accuracy. This includes such things as letting the person know that the record will be checked for accuracy, reinforcing accuracy in recording, asking the patient to monitor observable behaviors, recording as frequently and as close to the time of the behavioral occurrence as possible, using simple and accessible recording materials, and training the patient in how to self-monitor.

For the child who is unable to do self-monitoring, direct observation by the family members is a reasonable option. Indeed, this is probably the least used measure. Given that family members can become reliable observers and recorders, this system could provide a great deal of information on medication-taking behaviors.

The interview, another form of self-report measure, is probably the most commonly used measure in clinical practice and offers the advantages of identifying a portion of the noncompliers in a simple and inexpensive fashion. As well, it allows an in-depth review of the problems the noncomplier is encountering in carrying out the regimen. However, compliance tends to be overestimated with this measure, particularly if the patient has any degree of variability in medication-taking or -administering behaviors.

The pill count has become an alternative measure to the self-report. Pill counts are used commonly with adults and less often in the pediatric population. Where they have been utilized, they have not been reported. The pill count does provide a simple and inexpensive assessment of the extent to which an individual has complied with his regimen. It has the disadvantage of yielding an overestimate of compliance. The reliability of this method depends on the patient's willingness and ability to return unused medication for counting. This is particularly problematic if medication gets stored in various places or gets carried about during the course of the day. The pediatric studies that were noted to have utilized a pill-count method of assessment conducted these assessments in the home. While this may yield a more reliable measure than one would get from asking patients to bring unused medications into the clinic, it does add a measure of expense to the assessment procedure. Pill counts tend to have a fairly low correlation with the biological indices. However, as noted previously, the biological indices assess whether or not any medication was consumed in a relatively specific period of time, while the pill count gives an assessment of the degree of compliance over time. Further, the pill count will not identify the erratic medication taker, a problem that is more appropriately addressed by the various self-report measures.

An assessment procedure that is not yet in common usage is the mechanical monitor. Efforts have been underway to develop monitors that would measure compliance with such medications as bronchodilators and hypertensive medications. To date, these have been primarily experimental and have not been used in clinical practice. As interest increases and costs decrease, we may see more and more studies make use of the ongoing, daily, unobtrusive measurement that can be undertaken by the use of these mechanical devices, which both dispense and record the dispensing of various medications.

If one were to select a measure for compliance, it would be most useful to select a combination of measures that would serve to supplement the information that the others provided. One choice would be some form of direct observation or self-monitoring to offer information on the daily behavior surrounding compliance. Added to this would be an interview to obtain more in-depth information on the types of problems and successes encountered in consuming medication or administering it to a child. Third, in those cases where there is a question about medication consumption, the biological indices may be useful to determine if the drug or its metabolites are present and to what degree.

It should be kept in mind that, in addition to offering somewhat different information on compliance, the actual determination of the degree of compliance may vary with each measure (see Table 8.3). In the studies reviewed, the biological measures were the most common. Among these, the lowest compliance rates were found for the saliva assessment of bronchodilators (Eney & Goldstein, 1976). Higher rates were reported using serum indicators (Radius et al., 1978; Sublett, Pollard, Kadlec, & Karibo, 1978). Random unannounced urine assessments for antimicrobial activity also tended to report lower rates of compliance than routinely scheduled urine assays (36 to 40.1 percent versus 57.6 to 80 percent respectively) while the broadest range of response seems to come from the interview (18 to 87.9 percent). By examining this table, we can see that measurement method needs to be taken into account when compliance rates are examined.

Table 8.3
Measures of Medication Compliance

Drug	Compliance Measures	Author/Year	Compliance Range (%)
Antibiotics	Interview	Gordis et al. (1969b) Litt et al. (1980)	18–87.9
	Home pill count	Gordis et al. (1969b)	24–51
	Urine sample	Colcher & Bass (1972) Gordis et al. (1969a) Gordis et al. (1969b) Meyers et al. (1975)	57.6–80
	Random/un- announced urine sample	Buchanan & Mashigo (1977)	36–40.1
Anticonvulsants	Serum	Dawson & Jamieson (1971) Freiman & Buchanan (1978)	25–58
Bronchodilators	Saliva	Eney & Goldstein (1976)	11
	Serum	Radius et al. (1978) Sublett et al. (1979)	24.5–66.3
Chemotherapy	Urine sample	Smith et al. (1979)	41–82
Contraception	Interview	Litt et al. (1980)	44.6

Factors Associated with Noncompliance

Just who are the patients who fail to comply adequately with their treatment regimens? There seems to be no telltale characteristic. Indeed, any patient can relapse during the course of treatment; however, the literature in pediatric compliance has identified a few characteristics that may raise the clinicians' or researchers' alertness to potential pediatric compliance problems. These are:

1. Unmet expectations
2. Satisfaction with care
3. Lack of consequences for noncompliance
4. Side-effects (e.g., weight gain, skin changes)
5. Degree to which normal function is interrupted
6. Perception of the seriousness of the illness

7. Perceived likelihood of keeping child on the regimen
8. Perceived lack of control over recurrence
9. Large number of siblings
10. Older child (e.g., adolescent)
11. Clinic versus private practice
12. Attention getting
13. Parent management (weight loss)
14. Inadequate instruction
15. Pharmaceutical errors

The interaction with the health care provider seems to be critical. If the parents' expectations go unmet in the interaction, they are less likely to comply with the physician's advice (Francis et al., 1969; Korsch & Negrete, 1972). Similarly, the parent who is dissatisfied with care seems less likely to comply with the pediatrician's recommendations (Korsch & Negrete, 1972).

The consequences of compliance and noncompliance also appear to be important. Patients who experience an episode of noncompliance with no negative health consequences may be more likely to repeat their noncompliance. This has been noted in the case of diabetic children who have gone off their diets, have experienced no negative consequences, and subsequently have adhered poorly to their dietary regimen (Polowich & Elliott, 1977). With adults, side-effects when the patient has been compliant have not been associated strongly with noncompliance; however, this does not seem to be the case in the pediatric literature. Adolescents on steroid therapy for leukemia or following renal transplant—who experience such side-effects as weight gain, skin changes, and increases in irritability—tend to be noncompliant, even life-threateningly so (Korsch, Fine, & Negrete, 1978; Smith, Rosen, Trueworthy, & Lowman, 1979). Similarly, the degree to which the child's normal function or normal developmental behavior is interrupted seems to be associated with noncompliance (Gordis, Markowitz, & Lilienfeld, 1969c; Polowich & Elliott, 1977; Summey, 1978).

The experience of the parent also contributes to the degree of compliance. The mother's perception of the seriousness of the child's illness, as well as her perception of her likelihood of keeping the child on the regimen, are associated with parental noncompliance (Becker, Maiman, Kirscht, Haefner, & Drachman, 1977). Similarly, the mother's perception of a lack of control over the recurrence of the child's illness has been associated with noncompliance (Radius, Becker, Rosenstock, Drachman, Schuberth, & Teets, 1978). Gordis et al. (1969c) found that large families were related to noncompliance episodes, hypothesizing that the mother, overwhelmed by family responsibilities, may not be able to give the same time and attention to the child's medication as the mother in the smaller family.

Age also has been associated with compliance in the pediatric group; however, the direction is not consistent. Gordis et al. (1969c), Litt, Cuskey, & Rudd (1980), and Smith et al. (1979) reported lower rates of compliance among older children and adolescents than among younger groups of children. However, in the weight-management area, older adolescent girls tended to lose and maintain weight loss at a better rate than younger girls (Harris, Sutton, Kaufman, & Carmichael, 1980). Age may be moderated by the type of regimen that the child is on, as well as other factors. Children who are seeking attention from other adults or peers also may be noncompliant and, further, may falsify their own self-reports of compliance. In the case of children with diabetes, they may go so far as to falsify their urine-test reports (Simonds, 1979). In the weight area, children for whom the parent is managing the weight-loss regimen seem to regain weight more quickly than children who have a major responsibility for regulating their weight-loss program (Cohen, Gelfand, Dodd, Jensen, & Turner, 1980).

Factors specific to the delivery of health care also influence compliance. Shope (1981) notes in a review of pediatric compliance that clinic patients tend to adhere more poorly than patients seen in the private-practice setting. Other factors more specific to the health care providers include giving adequate instruction to the parent or the child (Sublett, Pollard, Kadlec, & Karibo, 1979) and making various pharmaceutical errors. For example, in a study conducted by Mattar, Markello, & Yaffe (1975), it was noted that among the sample of 100 patients there was 15 percent underfilling of antibiotic prescriptions at the pharmacy. Further problems occurred with misleading labels, which directed the patient to take medication too few times per day. A further problem is that the directions may advise the patient to take one or more teaspoons of medication a day, and yet there is great variation in the quantity that a household teaspoon actually holds (Allen, 1977; Mattar et al., 1975). Thus, the factors associated with compliance are not simply parent–child specific but also include problems associated with the direct provision of health care by professionals.

Intervention Studies in Compliance

The associated factors are a mixture of remediable and fixed problems. The question of what might be done to improve the care of children by improving their compliance rates is an interesting one, and, indeed, a few studies

Table 8.4
Intervention Studies with Pediatric Populations

Author/Year	Problem	Treatment	Intervention	% of Sample Compliant (Intervention vs. control)
Fink et al., 1969	Acute problems	Medications, varied	Nurse follow-up	59 vs. 18
Dawson & Jamieson, 1971	Epilepsy	Phenytoin	Increased supervision Drug monitoring: serum	80 vs. 25
Eney & Goldstein, 1976	Asthma	Theophylline	Drug monitoring: saliva	42 vs. 11
Mattar et al., 1975	Otitis media	Antibiotics	Education on regimen Drug calendar Dispensing device	51 vs. 8.5
Lima et al., 1976	Infections	Antibiotics	Reminders	59, 57 vs. 24
Colcher & Bass, 1972	Streptococcal pharyngitis	Penicillin	Schedules Parent counseling	80 vs. 50
Becker et al., 1977	Obsesity	Diet	Fear arousal	-2.5, -1.5 vs. 0 (% initial weight lost)
Magrab & Papadoulou, 1977	Renal dialysis	Diet	Token economy (inpatient)	0.97 lb. vs. 2.18 lb. gained between dialysis episodes

have attempted to do just that (see Table 8.4). These studies have utilized such methods as increased supervision, drug monitoring, education, drug calendars or dispensing devices, reminders, increased parent counseling and scheduling, fear arousal, and a token economy. A discussion of these studies follows.

Increased Supervision. Two studies have shown positive effects on compliance with increases in supervision. In the first case, Fink, Malloy, Cohen, Greycloud, & Martin (1969), in a medical center pediatrics clinic, examined the effectiveness of public-health nurses as family management specialists. Two hundred and seventy-four children were assigned randomly either to usual care or to the increased supervision offered by a nurse follow-up condition. Compliance was seen in 59 percent of the nurse-followed group, as contrasted with 18 percent of the control group. Similarly, Dawson & Jamieson (1971) examined the effect of increased supervision by increasing office visits until therapeutic blood levels of anticonvulsant medication were reached, and then they combined this process with routine monitoring of serum levels. Thirty children, ages six months to 12 years, were included in the study. There were no controls; all children were in the active intervention. Among this group, however, compliance was raised from 25 percent at the beginning of the intervention to 80 percent by the end of the six-month treatment period. Taken together, these studies suggest that increased supervision by the health care provider may be an important factor in raising the compliance rate among the population of pediatric patients who are having difficulties managing their regimen.

Drug Monitoring. Monitoring of medication taking or its effects in combination with either supervision or intervention also may be a useful strategy for improving compliance. As noted in the Dawson & Jamieson (1971) study, serum levels of anticonvulsant medication were monitored in the office setting, in addition to the increased supervision. Eney & Goldstein (1976) also evaluated the effect of biological monitoring, examining salivary levels of theophylline combined with increased supervision, using randomly chosen children with chronic asthma. One group of children was monitored with compliance in 11 percent of the group. A second group, whose members were told they would be monitored for compliance, had a 42% compliance rate. Thus, it seems that, while monitoring may have an effect, that effect may be stronger if the patients know they're going to be monitored. It should be noted, however, that in this case the groups were run sequentially, so a direct comparison cannot be made between the two. The results, however, are suggestive.

Mattar et al. (1975) also examined monitoring. In this case, the monitoring was of medication-taking behavior itself, in combination with a variety of other components in a package program. The multicomponent program consisted of verbal and written instructions for the administration of an antibiotic, a calibrated measuring device to overcome the problem of measurement variability in teaspoons, and a calendar to record doses taken. The effect of this package was tested for its compliance in children with otitis media. Thirty-three patients were studied through a hospital pharmacy and compared with 200 children who were going to neighborhood drugstores. The compliance rate in the multicomponent program was 51 percent as contrasted with 8.5 percent of the children going to neighborhood drugstores. Again, the study is not a carefully controlled, randomized trial; however, as with the preceding study, the results are interesting and suggest further investigation.

Reminders.   Since patients may report forgetting as a problem in complying with their medication regimen, Lima et al. (1976) investigated the use of reminders as a compliance-enhancing strategy with both adults and children on a short-term antibiotic regimen. Among the pediatric population, patients were divided into three groups. The first group was assigned to usual care. The second group received a clock-reminder prescription label. The parent was asked about usual routines; convenient times for taking the medication were circled on the clock on the prescription label. The third group received the same unique prescription label and, in addition, a refrigerator sticker reminding the parent to administer the medication. Twenty-four percent of the children in the usual-care group were judged compliant, that is, they exceeded 70 percent adherence by pill count. Fifty-seven percent of the children in the prescription-label-reminder group and 59 percent of the prescription-label-reminder plus refrigerator-sticker group were judged adherent. It would appear from this nicely controlled study that reminders may serve to enhance compliance over the usual sort of instruction offered.

Schedules and Parent Counseling.   Colcher & Bass (1972) also studied compliance-enhancing strategies with patients on antibiotics. In this case, the patients had streptococcal pharyngitis. The patients were assigned randomly to (1) a usual-care group, which was informed about medication taking in the usual manner, or (2) to a parent-counseling group, in which the parents were informed optimally on giving medication and were supplied with written instructions. Urine assay at the ninth day of treatment indicated that 50 percent of the patients in the usual-care group were compliant, while 80 percent of patients in the optimally informed, parent-counseling group were compliant. This study suggests that instruction of parents in how to carry out the regimen can increase compliance. Moreover, the written instructions given to the parents may have served as a reminder similar to the reminder offered by Lima et al. (1976) to parents in that study. Certainly, the use of reminder instructions and enhanced education are reasonable avenues for intervention.

Fear Arousal. Becker et al. (1977) examined the effect of fear arousal on weight loss in obese children. One group of children was given a high-fear message in a book about weight loss. A second group of children was given a lower-level of threat through their booklet, and a third group had no intervention at all. Becker and his colleagues reported greater weight loss in the high-fear group. This is not to suggest that fear-arousal strategies form a reasonable approach to all compliance-enhancing programs. Evidence in the adult compliance literature suggests that fear arousal may have negative effects on patients, leading them to feel helpless and overwhelmed by their condition and contributing, in fact, to noncompliance. It is likely that the arousal of some degree of anxiety regarding the health problem is important in motivating the patient to stay with the regimen, but high levels of arousal may, in fact, be dysfunctional.

Token Economy. Each of the preceding studies was completed in an outpatient setting. The one inpatient study was carried out by Magrab & Papadoulou (1977), who investigated the effect of an inpatient token economy on the minimization of weight gained through increased fluid intake in four young subjects between renal dialysis episodes. Weight gain was minimized during the token economy program, averaging less than one pound. When weight gain was withdrawn from the contingency system, weight gain averaged somewhat more than two pounds. This study suggests that, on the inpatient unit, the token economy system may be one strategy for inducing compliance.

Conclusions. Of these eight intervention studies, four used randomized control-group design (Fink et al., 1969; Lima et al., 1976; Colcher & Bass, 1972; Becker et al., 1977). Thus, considerable room remains for designing and evaluating intervention strategies to enhance compliance among the pediatric population. The few studies available suggest that relatively simple and inexpensive means may be used to improve compliance rates, although, even at best, the rates reach only 50 percent to 80 percent. These strategies include increased supervision on the part of the health care providers; drug monitoring, either through monitoring of biological indices or through self-monitoring using calendars; the provision of reminders; and the enhancement of parent education. Indeed, if one were to put together an adherence-improvement program, it would include such elements as a prescription compatible with the patient's and parents' lifestyle, clear communication and instructions regarding the regimen, written instructions and reminders, the introduction of a monitoring system (either behavioral or biological or both), and attention to close follow-up and supervision.

Suggestions for Future Research

There is still much to learn about the problems of pediatric compliance, as the gaps in this chapter certainly point out. First, we have much to learn about the extent of the problem of noncompliance in the pediatric group. This is particularly the case when we consider the inconsistent definitions for compliance, the arbitrary cutoff points for determining good adherence, and the variability in compliance rates, given differences in measurement procedures. Second, we still have much to learn about the factors that affect compliance in the pediatric population. It is not the case that parents are reluctant to give children medication. Indeed, in a study by Haggerty & Roghmann (1972) it was found that, over the 41,000 child-days studied, in 21 percent of those days at least one medication was administered to the child, and on an additional 3 percent of days two or more medications were administered. The authors of this study noted that the probability for a doctor contact on any given day is only 1 percent to 2 percent, and yet medication is administered on 26 percent of the days. So the problems that affect compliance go beyond the parents' willingness or ability to administer medication to the child. Factors that affect the parent as well as those specific to the child and the regimen need to be addressed. Differences between compliance rates, if such exist, in chronic and acute conditions, need to be examined. And the factors that differ between the compliance of children and compliance of adolescents need to be examined. Further, very limited research is available on the efficacy of interventions designed to remedy compliance problems. The studies that have been undertaken have addressed primarily parental problems. Certainly additional research needs to be done at this level, as well as research directed to the child and the specific regimen. Intervention studies also may be designed for the clinic or practice as well as various health care providers.

Summary

The state of knowledge of pediatric compliance is indeed in its infancy. We know that problems exist, and, based on the best evidence available, the problems seem to be relatively substantial. They cut across conditions and treatments and patient population groups. Our knowledge of the extent of these problems is handicapped by our inconsistent use of definitions and by measurement procedures. Even so, a number of factors have been identified that seem to be associated with patient noncompliance among the pediatric set. Some factors are remediable, others fixed; but considerable research is necessary to validate these findings as well as to determine the effect of remediating certain factors on subsequent compliance. Research also has begun on the identification and evaluation of strategies for enhancing compliance. If any area is open to further research, it is this one.

References

Allen, P. B. Pediatric patient compliance. *American Journal of Hospital Pharmacy,* March 1977, *34,* 229–231.

Arnhold, R. G., Adebonojo, F. O., Callas, E. R., Callas, J., Carte, E., & Stein, R. C. Patients and prescriptions: Comprehension and compliance with medical instructions in a suburban pediatric practice. *Clinical Pediatrics,* November 1970, 9:11, 648–651.

Barkin, S. Z., Barkin, R. M., & Roth, M. L. Immunization status: A parameter of patient compliance. *Clinical Pediatrics,* September 1977, *16*:9, 840–842.

Becker, M. H., Drachman, R. H., & Kirscht, J. P. Predicting mothers' compliance with pediatric medical regimens. *Medical Care,* October 1972, *81*(4), 843–854.

Becker, M. H., Maiman, L. A., Kirscht, J. P., Haefner, D. P., & Drachman, R. H. The health belief model and prediction of dietary compliance: A field experiment. *Journal of Health and Social Behavior,* December 1977, *18,* 348–366.

Buchanan, N., & Mashigo, S. Problems in prescribing for ambulatory black children. *South African Medical Journal,* July 1977, *52,* 227–229.

Cohen, E. A., Gelfand, D. M., Dodd, D. K., Jensen, J., & Turner, C. Self-control practices associated with weight loss maintenance in children and adolescents. *Behavior Therapy,* January 1980, *11*:1, 26–37.

Colcher, I. S., & Bass, J. W. Penicillin treatment of streptococcal pharyngitis: A comparison of schedules and the role of specific counseling. *The Journal of the American Medical Association,* November 1972, *222*:6, 657–659.

Dawson, K. P., & Jamieson, A. Value of blood phenytoin estimation in management of childhood epilepsy. *Archives of Diseases in Childhood,* June 1971, *46*:247, 386–388.

Eney, R. D., & Goldstein, E. D. Compliance of chronic asthmatics with oral administration of theophylline as measured by serum and salivary levels. *Pediatrics,* April 1976, *57*:4, 513–517.

Fink, D., Malloy, M. J., Cohen, H., Greycloud, M. A., & Martin, F. Effective patient care in the pediatric ambulatory setting: A study of the acute care clinic. *Pediatrics,* June 1969, *43*:6, 927–935.

Francis, V., Korsch, B. M., & Morris, M. J. Gaps in doctor–patient communication. *The New England Journal of Medicine,* March 1969, *280*:10, 535–540.

Freiman, J., & Buchanan, N. Drug compliance and therapeutic considerations in 75 black epileptic children. *The Central African Journal of Medicine,* July 1978, *24*:7, 136–140.

Gordis, L., Markowitz, M., & Lilienfeld, A. M. Studies in the epidemiology and preventability of rheumatic fever. Part IV. A quantitative determination of compliance in children on oral penicillin prophylaxis. *Pediatrics,* February 1969, *43*:2, 173–182. (a)

Gordis, L., Markowitz, M., & Lilienfeld, A. M. The inaccuracy in using interviews to estimate patient reliability in taking medications at home. *Medical Care,* January–February 1969, 7:2, 49–54. (b)

Gordis, L., Markowitz, M., & Lilienfeld, A. M. Why patients don't follow medical advice: A study of children on long-term antistreptococcal prophylaxis. *The Journal of Pediatrics,* December 1969, 75:6, 957–968. (c)

Haggerty, R. J., & Roghmann, K. J. Noncompliance and self-medication: Two neglected aspects of pediatric pharmacology. *Pediatric Clinics of North America,* February 1972, *19*:1, 101–115.

Harris, M. B., Sutton, M., Kaufman, E. M., & Carmichael, C. W. Correlates of success and retention in a multifaceted, long-term, behavior modification program for obese adolescent girls. *Addictive Behaviors,* January 1980, 5:1, 25–34.

Korsch, B. M., Fine, R. N., & Negrete, V. F. Noncompliance in children with renal transplants. *Pediatrics,* June 1978, *61*:6, 872–876.

Korsch, B. M., & Negrete, V. F. Doctor–patient communication. *Scientific American,* August 1972, *227*:2, 66–74.

Lima, J., Nazarian, L., Charney, E., & Lahti, C. Compliance with short-term antimicrobial therapy: Some techniques that help. *Pediatrics,* March 1976, *57*:3, 383–386.

Litt, I. F., & Cuskey, W. R. Compliance with medical regimens during adolescence. *Pediatric Clinics of North America,* February 1980, 27:2, 3–15.

Litt, I. F., Cuskey, W. R., & Rudd, S. Identifying adolescents at risk for noncompliance with contraceptive therapy. *The Journal of Pediatrics,* 1980, *96*:4, 742–745.

Magrab, P. R., & Papadoulou, Z. L. The effect of a token economy on dietary compliance for children on hemodialysis. *Journal of Applied Behavior Analysis,* Winter 1977, *10*:4, 573–578.

Markowitz, M., & Gordis, L. A mail-in technique for detecting penicillin in urine: Application to the study of maintenance of prophylaxes in rheumatic fever patients. *Pediatrics,* January 1968, *41*:1, 151–153.

Mattar, M. E., Markello, J., & Yaffe, S. J. Pharmaceutic factors affecting pediatric compliance. *Pediatrics,* January 1975, *55*:1, 101–108.

Meyers, A., Dolan, T. F., & Mueller, D. Compliance and self-medication in cystic fibrosis. *American Journal of Disease of Children,* September 1975, *129*, 1011–1013.

Polowich, C., & Elliott, M. R. The juvenile diabetic: In or out of control? *The Canadian Nurse,* September 1977, *73*, 24–27.

Radius, S. M., Becker, M. H., Rosenstock, I. M., Drachman, R. H., Schuberth, K. C., & Teets, K. C. Factors influencing mothers' compliance with a medication regimen for asthmatic children. *The Journal of Asthma Research*, April 1978, *15*:3, 133–149.

Shope, J. T. Medication compliance. *Pediatric Clinics of North America*, February 1981, *28*:3, 5–21.

Simonds, J. F. Emotions and compliance in diabetic children. *Psychosomatics*, August 1979, *20*:8, 544–551.

Smith, S. D., Rosen, D., Trueworthy, R. C., & Lowman, J. T. A reliable method for evaluating drug compliance in children with cancer. *Cancer*, January 1979, *43*:1, 169–173.

Sublett, J. L., Pollard, S. J., Kadlec, G. J., & Karibo, J. M. Noncompliance in asthmatic children: A study of theophylline levels in a pediatric emergency room population. *Annals of Allergy*, August 1979, *43*, 95–97.

Summey, P. S. Compliance of schoolchildren in getting and wearing glasses. *The Sightsaving Review*, Summer 1978, *48*:2, 59–69.

Wood, H. F., Feinstein, A. R., Taranta, A., Epstein, J. A., & Simpson, R. Rheumatic fever in children and adolescents: A long-term epidemiologic study of subsequent prophylaxis, streptococcal infections, and clinical sequelae. Part III. Comparative effectiveness of three prophylaxis regimens in preventing streptococcal infections and rheumatic recurrences. *Annals of Internal Medicine*, February 1964, *60*:2, 31–46, suppl.

Index

Abdominal pain syndrome, recurrent, *see* Recurrent abdominal pain (RAP) syndrome
Adrenocorticotropic hormone (ACTH), 109
Advertising, early smoking habits and, 137
Agarwal, V. K., 17
Alexander, A. B., 41, 46, 47, 52, 55, 57
Alexander, F., 38
Alexander, J. W., 78
Allergy shots, 37–38
Alluisi Performance Battery, 83–85
American Cancer Society, 140
American Health Foundation, 150
American Heart Association, 68
American Hospital Association, 108
Anderson, D. E., 92
Angelakos, E. T., 80
Antihypertensive drug therapy, 89–90
Aphonia, 114
Apley, John, 14, 15, 16, 17, 20, 21, 22, 23
Aragona, J., 197
Asthma, 28–66
  assessment in applied research, 44–45
  behavioral methods in treatment of, 46–60
  description of the asthmatic, 29
  incidence of, 28

  medical aspects of, 30–38
  psychological aspects of, 38–44
  scope of, 28
Asthma panic, 54–55
Asthmogenic allergens, 30
Asthmogenic stimuli, 30–32
Automobile accidents, 5
Aversive stimulation
  biological reactions to, 109–111
  controllability of, 108–109
  mitigation, 111–112
  pediatric hospitalization and, 112–114
  predictability of, 108–109

Baer, P. E., 80
Bain, H. W., 14
Barnett, P. H., 80
Barr, R. G., 15, 24
Bartel, A. G., 75
Bartlett, P. C., 80
Basal blood pressure, 67–68
Behavioral methods in treatment of asthma, 46–60
  alteration of asthma-related behaviors, 53–60
  alteration of pulmonary physiology, 46–53
Behavioral pediatrics, 1–12
  alternative clinical models for, 25
  automobile accidents and, 5
  behavior problems, 6–10

231

(*continued*)
　burns and, 6
　infections and, 6
　morbidity and mortality, 3–6
　pediatric practice, 2–3
Behavioral problems in clinical recurrent abdominal pain, 18–19
Behavioral programs for obese children, 187–200
Behavior problems, 6–10
　ranked for three-year-old boys and girls, 7
Berenson, G. S., 71, 77
Bergman, A. B., 2
Beta adrenergic blockage, 32
Beta-blocking agents, 89–90
Biesbroeck, R., 76
Biofeedback
　asthma and, 43
　elevated blood pressure and, 92–94
　relaxation and, 46–50
Biological factors, early smoking habits and, 141
Bires, J. A., 2, 6
Biron, P., 78
Blatter, M. M., 6
Bleecker, E. R., 41
Blendis, L. M., 21
Blood pressure, elevated, 67–106
　correlates among young persons of, 72–85
　measuring blood pressure in children and adolescents, 69–72
　research needs, 86–89
　treatment of, 89–99
Blood pressure reactivity, 68
Bloody stools, 14
Bogalusa Heart Study (1980), 69, 70, 71, 77–78, 82, 84
Bonk, C., 52
Borkowf, S., 8
Bortner Rating Scale, 82
Boulton, T. J., C., 76
Bourianoff, C. G., 80
Bradycardia, 90
Brand, R. J., 81
Breitrose, H., 78

Brody, K., 39
Bronchial asthma, *see* Asthma
Bronchodilators, 28, 60
Bronchospasm, conditioned, 42
Brown, B. W., 78
Bulimia, 185
Burns, 6

Calabrese, E. J., 77
California, University of (San Francisco), 87
Cardiovascular Research Institute, 87–88
Cardoso, R., 57
Cassady, J., 197
Cathode-ray terminal, 83
Chai, H., 39, 41, 47, 48, 52, 57, 58
Children's Manifest Anxiety Scale, 119
Child with Abdominal Pains, The (Apley), 16
Ching, A. Y. T., 40
Christensen, M. F., 14, 15, 22
Christophersen, E. R., 2, 5, 9
Clarke, P. S., 40
Clarke, W. R., 71
Coates, T. J., 69, 76
Comstock, G. W., 75
Conditioned responses, asthma and, 41–42
Cooper, A. J., 51
Cooper, B., 28
Coping behaviors, asthma and, 60
Corcoran, A. C., 78
Cornell University Medical College, 150
Coronary heart disease (CHD), 86
Corticosteroids, 28, 37
　side effects of, 29
Cotzias, G. C., 78
Coughing, asthma and, 56–58
Counselling Leadership Against Smoking (project CLASP), 148, 149, 150, 151
Court, J. M., 76
Cozzetto, F. J., 14
Craig, K. D., 22